Contents
Preface

Block 1 - Getting started

Chapter 1 - Start with a purpose
Intrinsic and extrinsic motivation
Purpose statement

Chapter 2 - How to make habits
Reminder
Routine
Reward
Keystone habits
Common mistakes

Chapter 3 - Overcome your limiting beliefs

Chapter 4 - Living your dream

Block 2 - Preparation strategy

Chapter 5 - Where do you stand today?
School/University exams
Competitive exams

Chapter 6 - Subject knowledge
Attending classes
Other sources of knowledge

Chapter 7 - Processing

Chapter 8 - Retention

Chapter 9 - Distractions
Common distractions
General ways to avoid distractions
Concentration

Chapter 10 - How to study
Getting into study mode
Planning the study

Block 3-Exam strategy

Chapter 11 - What to expect in the exam

Chapter 12-Before the exam
Planning for exams
Pre-exam stress
Dealing with anxiety
Dealing with low performance
Depression
Fear of failure
Dealing with ill health
Scheduling the exam

Chapter 13 - How to write the exam
Answering subjective papers
Objective type – General Instructions
Objective -Specific type of questions

Question Selection

Chapter 14 - What to do after the exam?
One-time exam
Series of exams

Block 4 - Becoming the topper

Chapter 15 - Attitude
The good
The bad

Chapter 16 - Habits
Develop a morning routine
Develop a night routine
Other Useful Habits

Chapter 17-People
Family Disturbances
People you need

Preface

If there is one thing which I have done consistently for a major part of my life, it is studying. I have written innumerable exams of diverse types and still scored well in all of them. That would have never been possible without the constant guidance and support of my parents.

I therefore dedicate this book to my parents without whom I would have never reached this stage.

I didn't want all those hacks and strategies to remain with myself. Hence, I decided to write this book to ensure the hacks to reach a lot of students. When I could ace any exam, even you will be able to do it after reading this book.

All the best!

☐

Block 1 - Getting started

Remember the first day of school every year?

You are excited and make new resolutions like, "This year, I will study well". Every academic year begins with such self-made promises for majority of you. The new books, school bag, uniform - everything excites you. You are attentive in class like never. You come back home and do your homework diligently. A week passes by with the same enthusiasm. But soon, you no longer find it exciting. Before you know it, you are slacking and have settled into your normal routine.

You no longer look forward to going to school. Studying becomes a chore you want to run away from.

Why does that happen? How can you prevent that?

☐

Chapter 1 - Start with a purpose

After reading this chapter, you will learn

- Why you are not able to study
- What your purpose is

You come back home after a tiring day and lie on the couch. You either binge eat or watch television. You do it daily but still won't get bored. Why is that? It serves a purpose. Your deeper need - the need to feel entertained.

Your true deeper purpose then becomes to feel entertained every moment.

Now when it comes to exams, you know the end goal. It is to get good marks in exams. "Okay! So what?" You need to study to get good marks in the exam. "Okay! So what?"

All through the process you know that there are a certain set of tasks to be done to reach the end. You need to attend classes, gather material, study, remember, write the exam. But there is no entertainment anywhere. Everything seems to be a task which needs to be done out of compulsion. There is no fun element at all in it. For how long can you do a piece of work which is forced?

That is the reason why many students fail in the exam. There is no deeper need which is being satisfied. You do it for the heck of it. Anything which is done superficially does not last long. You paint the outside wall of your house this year. In the coming rainy season, it chips off. During next summer, it fades. The next year, it looks like it had been ages that it had been painted. That is what happens when you study because you are expected to and not want it from within.

How to deal with it?

It has got to do with the workings of the human brain. Just like your school has different departments for different functions, the brain also has different areas for different activities. The part of the brain which deals with understanding that you need to study, the rational part, is different from the part which craves for needs, the emotional part. When you force yourself to study, the emotional part which thinks its needs are more important is not letting the message to be passed to the rational part. So, what you need to do is acknowledge that you have syllabus to be completed and make friends with the emotional part of the brain. For that, a connection needs to be established between the desired future and the innate need. You need to focus on getting the connection to keep the motivation going, in order to top the exam. This changes your behaviour and your motive to study. The need which was demanding entertainment before, will now make studying as a priority.

Intrinsic and extrinsic motivation

A lot of students keep looking for motivation to study regularly. A poster/picture which reads out inspirational quotes or personal goals is an external motivation. You can stick it on your wall, but your eye is on constant lookout for what is different from before. When you are looking at it daily, it doesn't make any difference to the eye. It stops being a reminder.
You can use this as your desktop wallpaper or phone wallpaper or even take a print of it and stick it on the wall. Do let me know for how long it has motivated you.

Hard Work Beats Talent When Talent Doesn't Work Hard

You can attend motivation seminars, read books and watch inspirational movies. But nothing will help unless you feel it at depth. The external motivation dies the moment you stop the external feeder. When you are clear about what you want to achieve, you tend to work on it for longer periods of time or until the purpose is realized.

So, sit down and write the purpose of your goal or resolution and the consequences of not achieving it. On days that you feel like giving up, go back and read it.

Purpose statement

Write the list of reasons why you want to study and score well in the exam.
a)
b)
c)
d)
e)
f)
g)
h)
i)
j)

How many of the reasons are valid reasons?

For you to have a reality check, go through the below list.

- Your parents want you to study
- Your friends are doing well
- You want to be praised by everyone
- You know it is important but don't know why

Or whatever your external reasons are.

When you study for your parents, you will succeed only till they constantly monitor you through the reward and punishment system. Once they stop it, you will be purposeless in life. You perceive the time invested in studying as life wasted.

When you want others to consider you successful, you are using an outer scorecard. Even if you are studying well and if people stop praising you, will you stop studying? That will eventually happen when you do it for others. Don't give the control of your life to others.

"Studying is the only way to be successful in life." At least this was bought by students in the older generation. They believed in whoever told this. This generation points hands at Bill Gates and Mark Zuckerberg, the college dropouts. But what about Elon Musk and Jeff Bezos? They graduated from University of Pennsylvania and Princeton University. Even though Bill Gates and Mark Zuckerberg dropped out of college they did that from Harvard.

If your reason is "What else should I do in life apart from studying?", you are again forcing yourself into studying but not finding a purpose.

Many students go for higher studies only to regret later because their reason was not strong enough. The only reason they don't give up is because they invested a lot of money in it. If you are wealthy or don't care for money, that will also not serve as a motivation.

Your purpose should be something which is tied to your bigger goal in life.

If your purpose in life is to become a doctor, scoring good marks in school will help you not only in gaining the knowledge but also to learn the right study techniques for future.

If you have no bigger goals in life, there is one need every human has. It is the need to know the unknown. Everyone wants the cognitive closure. Hence the need to seek out information. Connect that need with the external act of studying. Then your life goal changes from "I want to be entertained every moment" to "I want to gain knowledge every moment".
☐

Chapter 2 - How to make habits

After reading this chapter, you will learn

- Science behind habits
- How to form your habits

In the last chapter, you saw that you need intrinsic motivation. But if you just have intrinsic motivation but don't know how to channel it, it is going to be a waste.

From the time you wake up till the time you go to school, are there a set of activities you do daily? Those are your habits. Now, the present habits you have, may or may not be contributing to your goal of studying. So you need to learn how to form habits to make studying a cake walk for you. There is a scientific formula for it as Charles Duhigg writes in his book, The Power of Habit - Reminder, Routine, Reward, Repeat.

Reminder

To start doing something every day, you need a reminder. You eat when you are hungry. Why do you do this? Because hunger acts as a reminder that it is time for you to eat. In a similar way, for every habit, you want to make, find a reminder. There are 5 types of reminders - Time, people, place, event, emotion.

1.Time

Assign a daily or weekly slot for your habit. This slot is the trigger for your habit. Till you form the habit, use a reminder for the time slot.

Habit	Time
Study	I study as soon as the clock strikes 7 PM
Go to coaching classes	I go on Tuesdays and Thursdays

2. People

As soon as you see a few people, a few emotions are triggered. Similarly, you can make habits when you meet people. You can find accountability partners or study partners. When you meet people, it is the trigger for your habit.

Habit	People
Homework	I write homework as soon as my mother comes home
Solve puzzles	I solve puzzles whenever I meet my cousin

3. Place

When you are in a place, you need to be reminded of the habit. For example, when you are at the church, you pray. The place tells you what is expected of you.

Habit	Place
Study	As soon as I am in my study room, I get into studying mode
Ask doubts	Whenever I am at the coaching center, I get my doubts cleared

4. Event

Just like a domino effect, an event has a power to keep other events rolling.

Habit	Event
Homework	As soon as I finish evening snacks, I will do my homework
Write mock tests	As soon as a chapter is done, I write a test

5. Emotion

An emotion has the power to remind you that not everything is fine. Usually emotions trigger bad habits but when channeled productively, they can do miracles.

Habit	Emotion
Study more	When I feel jealous of my friend scoring for better than me, I will study harder
Study list	When I feel low about my performance, I make a list of next steps to be done

Routine

Start the habit in the smallest way possible and then slowly increase it. Currently, if the routine is not the smallest task and it requires your willpower to execute it, then you might not make it into a habit. Break it into smaller parts and start with the smallest.

If you want to make studying a habit, start with the smallest task - open the book every day. Then read one paragraph a day and then proceed to a few pages a day.

Routine becomes a habit only when it is done in a sustainable way. To make the routine sustainable, you can start it as a 30-day challenge. A 30-day challenge does not mean that you quit after the designated period. It must be continued even after the 30 days. But the initial 30 days serve as an external motivation which eventually gets converted to a habit.

Reward

For working so hard in the Routine step, you need a reward for the routine to stay. Reward need not be giving yourself a treat each time. It can be something as small as praising yourself or putting a tick mark on your daily checklist or feeling happy about the positive effects of the habit in your life. Using the Habit Tracker applications on smartphones is one of the effortless ways to keep a track of your routines while being rewarded, simultaneously. If you don't own a smartphone, you can write it in a book or use Microsoft Excel to track it.

Date	Maths	Science	Tests
28/4/2018	Y	N	Y
29/4/2018	N	Y	N
30/4/2018	Y	N	N

Go ahead and make a list of habits you want to build. Prioritize two of them for the first one month preferably keystone habits.

Keystone habits

Keystone habits help you create a lot of other habits without much struggle. It is similar to building a concrete foundation which keeps the building strong. What are the keystone habits which might help you in building other habits?

1. Waking up early

Morning is the best time for your brain as it is active and fresh after a good night's sleep. It acts as a keystone habit as it helps you make time for

- Exercise
- Decision making

- Planning the day
- Preparing for the class
- Eating breakfast
- Solving complex problems

Common mistakes

Students make the following mistakes while making new habits

1.Start Big

When you start, you start it big. Because you want to achieve everything the first day itself. You are not to be blamed. It is your excitement. But when you start off that way, will you be able to sustain it?

Start so small that the routine doesn't feel like a routine at all. The task may be as big as reading the entire chapter. But start with just one definition the first day.

2.Not getting back after a miss

It is okay to miss your habits on a few days. But what matters is getting back to it after missing it. If it feels tough, you can start with the smallest task again. But get back and keep doing it.

3.Not increasing the pace

Once you are used to the smallest task, slowly increase the task in a reasonable pace. If you keep doing the smallest task, you might never reach your goal.

Chapter 3 - Overcome your limiting beliefs

After reading this chapter, you will learn

- Why you are not willing to put in efforts
- What is stopping you from making any progress

Do you know why an elephant, who is strong enough to pull up trees, doesn't try to flee when tied with a small chain? When the elephant was young, it was tied with a strong chain. It tried hard to escape, but it could not get rid of the chain. After a point, it started accepting that the chain cannot be gotten rid of. It slowly got habituated to listening to its master. This tiny event changed the purpose of its life. Hence, the gigantic animal has given up on its freedom and accepted its fate.

Are you any different from the elephant?

Have you seen beautiful birds that are caged and captive bred? These birds remind most of us of protagonists in the movies who free them up to show it off as an act of kindness. But, a bird which has been domesticated for so long will not know what to do with its freedom. It will not know how to protect itself from its predators. It can't search its own food because all its life it has only been fed. It is weaker compared to other birds of the same species because it was not taught how to live by itself.

Are you any different from the bird?

If you notice closely, your life is similar to the elephant and the bird. You were told that you were not capable of a few things. You just thought that it was true to the core because everyone said the same.

If you are shown what your problem areas are and are given the solutions to them, will you act right away?

No, you won't do that.

You believe deeply that you can't be changed. You think that nothing you do will bring any change.

You will feel that your identity is being changed if shown that you can become intelligent too.

Stop enjoying self-pity.

Even if you choose to agree or not, you are guilty of doing the above.

You want other people to sympathize with you that you can't study or remember beyond what you are doing right now.

But, you are a lot more capable than what you think you are. You need to let go off the beliefs which you are hoarding currently.

The beliefs can be anything from "I can't focus however hard I try" to "I can't get over my anxiety in examination hall".

Ponder over your belief systems and make a list of your limiting beliefs here.

_____
_____
_____
_____
_____
_____
_____
_____
_____

Whatever your issues are, they are all addressed in the coming chapters. All you need to do is be willing to let go off the beliefs, learn the techniques and embark on a new journey.

Chapter 4 - Living your dream

After reading this chapter, you will learn

- Why you are not able to study
- What your purpose is

When you look at studying as a chore, it is painful. But when you associate it with your dream, you will find the entire journey to be exciting.

1.You will no longer fear the future

If you are constantly worried about exams, you will never be at peace. You will always be worried.

"What if I did not get through the exam?"
"What if I don't get my dream college?"
"What if I am left behind?"

Worrying about things beyond your control is self-inflicted agony. Loving your dream and working towards it is self-assuring.

2.You will stop feeling inferior

When you don't perform well in exams due to unforeseen circumstances, the following scenario will make you feel inferior if your focus is only on marks.

Friend 1: "I stood first in class."
Friend 2: "I stood second in class."

This happens because you forget the purpose behind doing it. Instead, when you focus on the purpose, you are more connected to your goal and not scoring marks will not bother you anymore. The feeling of inferiority will then be gone.

3. You enjoy your day

You do not run after exams or wait for holidays. You enjoy today. Because you are doing what you believe in.

4. You don't need external motivation

Your routines are in place. You work in an auto-pilot mode. You don't have to push yourself to study daily. You do your tasks because you love the reward, they give you.

5. You feel smarter

When you are looking at the end goal, your vision is narrow. You soon forget what you read. But when you associate your goal with a purpose, it sticks with you for a lifetime. You grow as a person. Your goal nurtures you.

6. You become proactive

You don't leave your future to destiny. You anticipate problems and take preventive measures.

7. You feel more responsible

You don't blame the surroundings/situations. You take responsibility for the mistakes and correct them.

8. You will find your mentor

Mentors come to those who work on their dreams. When they see potential, they will catalyze the growth.

9. You don't feel overwhelmed by success or failure

You study for the satisfaction of it. You are not bogged down by the highs and lows in the tests.

10. You start feeling out of place

You no longer fit into a peer group. You will see your friends running after exams mindlessly. But, you will be calmer and more stable.

11. You will stop perceiving passive entertainment as a priority

Watching a TV show won't be a priority anymore. You know that it can wait and does not fit into the bigger purpose.

12. You won't have time to complain

You will then know that half the problems can be solved in the time spent on complaining and finding excuses.

13. People will start admiring you

It is not the reason why you should work on your dreams. But when you see someone doing something which you are not, you automatically start admiring them and vice versa.

14. You feel more contented

Above all, you go to sleep with a peaceful mind that the day has been spent well.

None of the above is possible if you don't have the mindset that studying is for the purpose and not for scoring marks alone.

Block 2 - Preparation strategy

Remember the sleepless nights you spent before the exam but could not recollect anything in the exam?

Do you find it difficult to focus when you sit to study?

You are interested in studying but don't know how to plan. Do you wish you had someone who can guide you?

Whatever your concerns are on approaching the subjects, this block is for you to know the strategy used by toppers to remember all the concepts.

Chapter 5 - Where do you stand today?

After reading this chapter, you will learn

- Your present performance levels
- Your problem areas

You are reading this book to improve your scores in exams. But how will you know if you have improved or not over the time?

You need to know where you stand today to know where you can reach tomorrow. To measure yourself, you don't have to take an IQ test. This book is not for improving your intelligence. But to show that you are intelligent, scoring wise.

There are two types of tests. One is the regular tests which you take at schools and colleges. The other is competitive tests. The topper of your class at school need not be the topper in competitive exams. Even if you have scored only 60% in school tests, you can be trained to score good percentile in competitive tests and vice versa.

Performance in School/University exams

What have your scores been so far?

This year _____

Last year _____

Two years back _____

Are they consistent?

a) Yes
b) No

Has there been an improvement or are they staggered?

a) Improvement
b) Staggered
c) Decrement

Is there a peak in your scores? What are the reasons for it?

_____
_____
_____
_____

Is there a dip in your scores? What are the reasons for it?

_____
_____
_____
_____

For example, let's look at the scores of a student

This year: 80%

Last year: 82%

Two years back: 90%

Are they consistent?

They have been consistent for the last two years. But he did better two years earlier.

Has there been an improvement or are they staggered?

He was good before, but I started scoring less since last year.

If there is one peak what are the reasons for it?

He put in extra efforts that year which he didn't earlier.

If there is one dip what are the reasons for it?

He was not able to spend so much time on studying for the past two years.

Do a similar analysis for your scores. The analysis can be done for different quarters in the same year too. This example is just to give you an idea on how to start with the performance analysis.

Now you get a rough idea of where you stand. Let's deep dive into your problem areas.

If you are not doing well, the problem lies either in

1.Interest

You are not interested in a subject or any subject at all. You are not interested in getting the formal education.

2.Other factors

You are interested and ready to put in effort but struggling to study. This happens due to

a) Lack of basics

Many students find it difficult to recollect the basics of a subject. When the basics are not strong, you will not be able to understand the advanced concepts at depth. Hence the retention suffers.

b) Lack of guidance

You don't know the right resources for the exam and lack a study plan.

c) Study habits

You might be using cramming as the method of studying instead of understanding the concepts. Maybe you are irregular with your studies or not focusing in the class.

d) Distractions

Your attention span is below par and can't focus for more than a few minutes.

e) Retention

You forget what you read a while ago.

f) Retrieval

You remember the concepts but can't retrieve it at a later point of time.

g) Unable to perform in exams

Even if you know the answers to all the problems in the paper, it is as useless as not knowing anything if you can't answer them.

So what are your problem areas?
a)
b)
c)
d)
e)
f)
g)

It can be one or more than one or all of them. Read the techniques in the following chapters to improve in all areas but focus more on your problem areas to see a stark improvement in your scores.

Performance in Competitive exams

These exams range from Olympiad tests at school level till entrance exams for higher studies or jobs. Before you start preparing for a competitive exam, either refer to a question paper from the previous year of the subject or take a mock test of that online. It gives you an idea of where you stand as of today.

Whatever you score in regular exams will not be a predictor for how you might score in competitive exams. If you are a just-before-exam crammer, you will score well in the internal subjective exams. For the external objective type exams, you need the concepts. If you are someone who likes studying the concepts in depth and doesn't care about marks in subjective exams, you will have an extra edge in the objective competitive exams.

Whatever might be the case, you hold a chance to improve and even top the exam by changing your strategy.

How much have you scored in the mock test? _____

What is the highest a topper can score on the same test?
_____

Let's say you scored 90 out of 100 in the exam and the paper was difficult. You thought you scored 90 percent in the exam. But what if the topper scored 91? Rest of the questions were too difficult to answer by others too in such a short span of time. So, the results in competitive exams are usually relative. You should not worry too much about your absolute score, but about how good or bad your absolute score is, when compared to others who took the same test.

Note:

Comparison of scores with toppers is mentioned here to account for relativity. But if the scoring is done in absolute terms, you need not bother about what others are scoring. Your aim should be to score full marks.

What problems did you encounter while solving the paper?

a) Lack of subject knowledge

If you are attempting the test for the first time, you would not be aware of the concepts to start with. Learning the concepts will help you overcome this problem.

b) Difficulty applying the subject knowledge

If you are thorough with the basics but find difficulty in applying the concepts, you would not have practised enough. This is relatively easier than the before problem because all you need to do is practice on how to apply the knowledge.

c) Stuck between two answer choices

You can eliminate a few options and stuck with two of them. Even though this is easiest of the cases, it is a bit tricky. But it can be dealt with by increasing the depth of your preparation.

d) Time management

If you are given unlimited time, you can solve the entire paper with no hassle. But in exam hall, you are not able to do it. If this your problem, all you need to do is learn question selection and other hacks of writing exam. It is more of smart work than hard work. You can easily learn this, too.

e) Focus

If you find it tough to sit in one place with single-minded attention, it is going to be an arduous task to do it for the first time in the exam hall. But it can be achieved by focussing during various mock exams.

f) Exam anxiety

If your mind goes blank due to nervousness, you should be glad that you diagnosed this problem at this stage. It takes quite a bit of time to deal with it and overcome it.

The hacks for problems a, b, e are explained in this block and for c, d, f are explained in the third block.

Fill the below:

Present score: _____
Desired score: _____

Problem areas
a)
b)
c)

d)
e)
f)

For Example, let's look at the values filled by a student.

Present score: 80
Desired score: 99

Problem areas
a) Subject knowledge
b) Exam anxiety

Now you are ready to start fixing your issues.

Chapter 6 - Subject knowledge

After reading this chapter, you will learn
- How to make the most of guided coaching
- Alternatives to classroom learning

The first step to acing exams is to acquire the knowledge required for the exams. This can be done in three ways – guided coaching, self-study and group study.

Classrooms

The default source of knowledge for school and college going students is through classes. It is the most traditional and conventional way of gaining knowledge.
A lot of students ask, "Why should I attend the class when they teach only from the textbook or read the slides?"

When should you attend classes?

This depends on various factors

1.Quality of lecture

One of the most deciding factors for attending any class is the quality of the lecture. The quality further depends on

a) The complexity of the subject

If you are being taught in a class which can be procured only by putting a lot of efforts to search from multiple knowledge sources, the class is a must attend. In fact, making notes becomes even more important in this scenario.

b) Delivery of the subject

If the subject is complex and the lecturer makes it fun by explaining the concept in layman's terms, it makes the lecture worth attending. Even if the lecture is delivered in a structured way, it makes the retention easier.

2. Compulsion of Attendance

If you are not eligible to attend the exams unless you attend the class, you have no other choice than to be in the class. When you are in the class, you are not going to lose anything in listening to the lecture even if the lecturer is going to read from the book or the slides. Getting hold of a few terminology or key phrases will help you build a story in the exam.

3. Concentration skills

If you haven't slept the entire night, you won't gain anything from waking up to an alarm and going in a half-sleep mode to class. You will end up fighting sleep or sleeping in class and gain nothing from the class. It will also deteriorate your health in the long run. Fix this problem first by following a regular sleep schedule.

If the lecture is interesting and if you are still not able to concentrate, go through the chapter 10 on how to study so that you will learn to develop an interest in the subject.

Where to sit in the class?

Even though a few research studies say that where you sit in the class does not matter, there are a few other research studies which say that sitting closer to the lecturer has a positive impact. It helps not only in being attentive and participating in class discussions but also in having a good peer group to discuss the subject.

If it is a subjective type of exam which will be evaluated by the same lecturer, there is a higher chance of the lecturer giving you good scores when you sit in his vicinity and actively participate in the class. Also, if you approach the lecturer outside class, there are higher chances of him mentoring you.

Usually, the backbenchers are those with low self-esteem who are not willing to pay much attention in class. Even if you are a bright student, you might lose out interest in the long run if there is disturbance around you all the time.

There are exceptions to this too. I was a backbencher in school since I was one of the tallest girls in the class but that never stopped me from paying attention in the class.

What to do before the class?

Go through the concepts of the topics that will be taught in the class the next day.

Even if you are an average student today, glancing through what you are going to learn will be helpful. It is like watching a trailer before you go to the movie. If you are already doing well in studies, it is advisable to study the topic by yourself before the teacher teaches you. The class acts like a filler for the gaps in your understanding which will help in stronger retention of the information.

How to do it?

If the class today is on the poem 'The road not taken' by Robert Frost, you need to be aware that a poem written by Robert Frost will be taught. Ask yourself questions like:

Did I come across this author before?

What could the title mean?

The poem could be about doing something unconventional in life.

Are there any new words in the poem?

A quick glance will tell you about them.

So, what you must be aware of will vary from subject to subject. The above example is to depict the approach you need to develop.

What to do in the class?

1.Listen attentively

This is the most obvious thing. But when it comes to implementation, it does not remain an obvious act anymore. If there is one thing which completely explains the strategy of toppers, it is listening with utmost attention. Being attentive in class itself gets half your work done.

2.Summarize

At the end of each class or whenever the lecturer pauses, summarize whatever he taught. There might be some gems in the explanation at his end and the understanding that has taken place at your end. You might forget this simplified version of the concept later.

3. Make mental movies

Note down the key points and map them in your mind in an interesting way. If the lecture is on the places in North America and their significance, visualize the same in your mind as lecturer shows it on the map.

4. Take notes

If you find it tough to concentrate in class, start taking running notes. You will feel forced to pay attention. Even if you are not able to comprehend it, when you refer to them later, you will not miss any points which were told in the class. This makes the time spent in attending lectures productive.

5. Solve problems

If it is a class which requires you to solve problems, don't peek into your friend's book. Do it by yourself. If you get stuck, confused or get the answer wrong, ask your teacher. He is the best person to guide you and clear your doubts. Half the learning happens in the class if you pay attention.

6. Ask doubts

If you don't understand something, get it clarified. If you understand everything, summarize it. Constantly interact with your teachers to map your progress.

7. Reply to questions

Most of the teachers try to make the class interactive. Be active and participate in the discussion. It is one of the ways to increase the attention and retention span.

What to do after the class?

Consolidate your entire learning in one sentence or a few keywords.

If the class was about World War I, write down the important years, dates, the starters of the war and how it ended.

The summary will look like
- 1914-1918
- Triple Alliance vs General Powers
- League of Nations

Should you attend additional classes?

This needs to be dealt with in two parts:

Part 1 - School and college

If your basics are weak or if you are not able to follow the classes given by your school or college teacher, going for additional classes where you are able to follow the teacher will be helpful. But then again, attending the classes alone will not be enough. You will have to put in efforts to reinforce the learning.

There are two types of additional classes:

1.Mass coaching

This is helpful only if your aim is to get subject knowledge from another source or if you want to make friends to form a study group. If they provide mock tests and constant feedback, even in that case it is going to be helpful.

2.Individual attention

If your basics are not strong, going for a mass coaching will be useless. You need a tutor who understands your shortcomings and teaches you from scratch. While you may find it a little more expensive than mass coaching, it will be beneficial in the long run if you work on your foundations. So, find a tutor who can fix your basics and logical thinking.

Part 2 - Competitive exams

Coaching institutes

You should go to a coaching center if you

- Have no idea of the subject
- Want a structured way of learning
- Are not confident about doing it yourself
- Want a study group
- Need a mentor

But going to a study centre alone won't make you an expert on the subject because coaching institutes do not have time to spend working on individual concerns. Consider joining study centres, only if your basics are strong and only need guidance on how to apply it effectively.

A lot of coaching institutes have the basic classes and leave the practice sessions to the students. It is not sufficient if you learn something for once in class. You need to revise it to make it permanent in your memory. It is not sufficient if you know that distance is the product of speed and time. You should know how to apply it. You will know it only if you practice it after going home.

For the subject knowledge to stick in your head, you need to put in additional efforts as well.

Online Classes

To complement your knowledge, you can choose to take courses online. MOOCs on Coursera, Edx, NPTEL are available for free. Khan Academy also explains a lot of concepts.

There are a lot of videos on the internet too. But you cannot predict their reliability. Even if there are a few faults in the video or the website you are referring to, it will cost you a lot.

Books

1.Study material

If you can't afford to attend formal schooling or go to a coaching centre or if it is not available in your locality, you must get the right study material. Instead of buying too many books and fretting that you are not able to complete the syllabus, rely either on official websites or friends who have access to formal coaching for the right study material.

If you can't afford to buy the material, you can

a) Buy it on a sharing basis

Get a friend to join you or make a group and buy books collectively. You can then make a schedule to share and use it as per your comfort.

b) Borrow the books

You can either borrow them from a library or book shops which lend.

c) Go to a library

If you can't afford any of the above, you can choose a library as your place of study.

Chapter 7 - Processing

After reading this chapter, you will learn

- How information is processed in the brain
- Different types of memories

When you first look at the information, it enters your brain as sensory data. If you are paying attention to it, it gets stored in the short-term memory. Now if your brain thinks that it is important, it will transfer it to long-term memory based on how your brain can make connections with it.

When your friend and you have been subjected to the same knowledge exposure, both of you don't retain the same level of information. It is not because of the source of information but based on how it is processed in each of your brains.

Even if you are present in class and listening to your teacher but looking at your crush, the information will not move into short-term memory. As you are reading this book now, you had been paying attention till now and the sensory information has been being transferred to your short-term memory. But after you saw the word crush, you have not stopped reading it and sensory signals have also been generated but they are no longer moving into your short-term memory because the previous sentence pulled out memories from your long-term memory about your crush. This caused a disruption in further processing. Instead, when you were reading about this cycle and could connect it with a similar concept you read before, your brain is already making connections with the long-term memory to remember how information processing works in the brain.

Let us learn more about this

Short-term memory

- It constantly interacts with the long-term memory
- It has low capacity. It can remember 7 plus or minus 2 numbers at a time. This is also called Millers number.
- The duration is very low may be less than 30 seconds
- It is the place where thinking and reasoning happens

Working memory

- Working on the information from short-term memory is called working memory
- All the thinking happens in this
- If this memory is loaded with too many activities at the same time, it is called cognitive load. The higher the cognitive load, the lower the productivity of your studies.

Connections

The main way to push the information from short-term to long-term memory is to form the connections. The tip which I mentioned in the previous chapter to prepare for the class before-hand works on this principle. It reduces the cognitive load since you are aware of what is going to be taught. Since you have been dwelling on the topic for a while now it will be easier to make the connections. This process is also called active learning since there is a constant exchange of information between the short-term memory and long-term memory.

A lot of students complain that they have a problem concentrating. But when you understand the above process, distraction can happen at multiple levels. The first part of distraction can be called selective attention. Paying attention to your crush or a notification on your smartphone makes you pay attention to an information which is not the desired information now. In the chapter on distraction, you can read about how you can correct this. The next part of distraction occurs when you are not able to transfer the information from short-term memory to long-term memory. This is mostly referred to by students as "I study but I don't remember," or "I am attentive in classes, but I can't recollect". This is dealt in the next chapter on retention.

Chapter 8 - Retention

After reading this chapter, you will learn

- Why you are not able to retain with your present study methods
- How to study smart

The retention methods which make you fail

a) Cramming

965789

If I ask you to remember this number, you are going to force it into your head. You keep repeating it, till you can remember it. If I ask you the same number tomorrow, you might not be able to recollect it. Cramming won't help you in any way because the content won't go into the long-term memory. It gets into your short-term memory through selective attention and can't find any content in the long-term memory to make connections with.

You can write and rewrite the subject to cram it up until your head is filled with nothing but knowledge about the chapter. But do you think that you can pull this off for an exam which has tons of material to read?

b) Rereading

Go back and read the previous chapter to teach your friend how the brain works. Are you able to recollect everything in order? You will fumble. Instead recollect it now and then go back and read the parts you can't recollect. Are you able to present it better that way?

Rereading without recollection in between is fooling yourself that you are studying hard. It makes you over learn it but not retain it. You will end up forgetting in the long term. Instead of reading it continuously, read it by giving enough spaces.

The retention methods which will not let you forget the concepts even after years

1.Get an idea

Anything which needs to be retained must undergo some amount of mental effort. In this chapter, we will see different ways in which we can increase the retention.

Research confirms that taking a quiz on a topic before learning about it helps in retaining it better.

Ask yourself what your expectations are from learning a subject or topic.

You don't have to go in search of pre-quizzes for a topic now. If you are going to study about earthquakes, write down a few pointers about what you already know about earthquakes. If you know nothing, you can try going by etymology. Earthquake is a quake of the earth which means that the earth shakes. Now pose some questions to yourself.

- What makes the earth shake?
- How do we feel it when it shakes?
- What will happen when the earth shakes?
- How to know if it is dangerous?
- What are the consequences of it?
- Can they be prevented?

If you feel you are incapable of posing any questions, just ask

- What
- How
- Why

- When

They always help.

Now when you attend the lecture, you will find answers to your questions.

By doing this

- You will feel interested in the subject
- You will fill the gaps in your knowledge
- You prepared the long-term memory ready to connect with the short-term memory

After the lecture, go back and write answers to the questions you posed for yourself.

2.Space your learning

Can I finish the entire subject in a day?

Yes, without a doubt.

The question you should ask yourself is can I remember the subject if I read it in one go?

According to a research study, 38 surgical residents were divided into two groups. They wanted to study 4 short lessons in microsurgery. One group thought they were smart and finished the entire subject in a day. The second group were a bit lazy and decided to do one lesson per week. But they were disciplined enough to stick to their schedule.

Now when they had to practice this on real rats, the first group performed terribly. They stumbled while performing the surgery. But the disciplined group was adept.

What did you learn from the story?

You are smart enough to do it all in one go. But become smarter and don't do it all in a day. Space it out.

What is the advantage of spacing out?

When you reopen the book after a week, you will find it difficult to recollect what you read last week. But the struggle you are putting yourself through is what makes the neurons stronger. The neurons need a lot of time to do their processing and consolidation.

You become strong only after you fall. If everything goes well, how will you ever learn the difficult part?

So do your neurons. They need to struggle to remain strong.

If you finish off the entire syllabus in one go, you are relying on your short-term memory and not letting it establish itself in the long-term one.
If I must take a gap for one week, what am I supposed to do for the rest of the week?
No. You are not playing. You are not watching TV. You are not involving yourself in gossip.
But you are going to read other subjects.

If in the first slot, you are reading subject A. In the second slot, read subject B. Then the third slot, do subject C. Now repeat the cycle. But don't go back to the same topic of subject A. Instead choose a different subtopic in A. Same with B and C.

Your normal schedule

9-10 AM Mathematics – Geometry
10-11 AM Physics – Rotational Mechanics
11-12 PM Chemistry - Organic

Break time

1-2 PM Mathematics – Geometry

2-3 PM Physics – Rotational Mechanics
3-4 PM Chemistry – Organic

Your revised schedule

9-10 AM Mathematics – Geometry
10-11 AM Physics – Rotational Mechanics
11-12 PM Chemistry - Organic

Break time

1-2 PM Mathematics – Arithmetic
2-3 PM Physics – Electromagnetic theory
3-4 PM Chemistry – Inorganic

This will help you to recollect effortlessly in the final examination hall.

3.Variety

a) Should I revise the same topic for an entire year?

Did you ever use www.vocabulary.com? It uses standard learning techniques to help you learn new words. So even if you are perfect with the concept, you need to retrieve it at periodic intervals for it to stick in the long-term memory.

b) How many problems of the same type should I do to become perfect in the concept?

Try these.

What number should I add both to the numerator and denominator of 4/5 to make the ratio 7/9?

What number should I add both to the numerator and denominator of 4/5 to make the ratio 11/12?

What number should I add both to the numerator and denominator of 4/5 to make the ratio 13/14?

Now in the exam, you are asked,
I am twice your age now. How many years back was I thrice your age? My present age is 28.

Do you feel tongue-tied?
Do you feel cheated?
Do you think the books, the lecturer and the examiner wanted to take revenge on you?
Weren't you the one who asked how many problems of the same type I should practice?
You practiced 3 problems of the same type. But when the question is twisted, you are confused and bewildered.
That is the reason why you should practice different types of problems instead of the same type.

Let's say your colleague applies oil to her hair, ties it in a bun for office uniform. One day, you happen to meet her outside and see her hair left out and in fashionable clothes and makeup. You might not be able to recognize her if not for her facial features.

That is how problems are too.

4.Homework

Should you take homework seriously?

Yes, dig into the purpose of it. When you don't see a purpose to the homework you don't have to do it.

Most of the time, the purpose of homework is to make you practice. When a lecturer teaches a new concept, he first teaches you the basics. Before increasing the depth of the topic, he wants you to be perfect with the basics. If you can't catch up with the pace, you are the one who will be at loss.

5. Making Notes

a) Don't make notes as sentences

Your brain does not remember individual words you read but the summary. When you make notes don't write the entire story. Write the one word which can help you recollect the entire chain of words which represent it.

Steam, hot, coal, burn, hot spring, boil.

Your brain does not remember them as individual words. But it just remembers as those words are related to being hot.

b) Use differences table wherever it is possible

Short-term memory

- It is like RAM
- Selective attention determines what enters into it
- Only 7 plus or minus 2 items can be remembered at a time

Long-term memory

- It is like hard disk
- It remembers based on importance
- Limits are unknown

Feature	STM	LTM
Computer component	RAM	Hard disk
Information entry	Selective attention	Importance
Limit	7 plus or minus 2	Unknown

Which one do you think is easier to remember?

c) Highlighting

Don't highlight the sentences. Highlight the keywords. The keywords you highlight should be able to tell the entire story of the chapter.

d) Where to take notes?

i) Margins:

Consolidate the entire page in a few words in the margin. So that next time you go through the book, you don't have the read the entire page.

ii) Loose sheets:

It is difficult to maintain the sheets. There are chances that you might lose them with rough work. But if you like writing in sheets only, maintain a file or folder to save them all categorically.

iii) Book:

It is advisable to have a separate notebook for each topic. Or else you can write one topic from the front and another topic from the back. If the book gets filled up soon, make sure that you number the books in proper order. There can't be worse cognitive load than searching for the right book. Make notes for the entire chapter in one book instead of writing different parts of the topic in different books. It will avoid wastage of time in compiling the information for revision.

iv) Online applications:

Keep:

If you want to remember in term of short pointers, Keep is a nice application.

It can be used more as a to-do list for the day than for writing notes. But the colors make them good flash cards.

Onenote:

If you are well versed with Windows, you can go for this app. It helps you organize notes in a structured manner. You can have multiple sub-branches under one notebook.

Evernote:

It has features similar to OneNote. You can first click on new Notebook and then add multiple text notes under it. The drawback of Evernote is that sub notes are not possible under this text note.

It is an excellent web clipping tool. If your studying requires clipping articles from the web, Evernote is the one to go for.

e) How to use pens while making notes?

Use different markers for different types of events while highlighting. While making notes too, try to use different colors to make it pleasant for you to read when you want to revise.

6. Mnemonics

When you must memorize facts, it is sometimes difficult to form connections. That is where memorization comes to your rescue.

a) Remembering numbers

Associate numbers with something you like. If you must remember 2515, it is a combination of birthdays of your mother and father. Not that it is this easy, but you can still find a funny way to remember.

b) Anagrams

If you must remember the colors of a rainbow, you have to remember the word VIBGYOR.

V - Violet
I - Indigo
B - Blue
G - Green
Y - Yellow
O - Orange
R - Red

c) Flashcards

Pictures are easier to remember. Associate words with pictures. Carry a flashcard of the picture. As soon as you see the picture, you can recollect the information associated with it.

If you can't find a picture, you can just use a keyword and write the definition on the back of it.

d) Mind maps

Write the central idea at the center. Draw out branches to talk about various characteristics of the central idea. The branches also should be in words and not detailed sentences.

e) Flowcharts

Represent the entire chapter as a flowchart. It tells you from where it started and where it ended. It is not only easy to read but also easy to retrieve.

f) Questions

Make notes as questions.

'Why? Where? When? How?' - These will help you set a question paper for yourself if you can't find mock tests.

g) Weave the words

Let us see a sample of this with 10 words.

Carrot
Man
Car
Feather
Bottle
Phone
Teacher
Love
File
Ring

To remember this list, weave a story with the words.

Carrot looks red. A man went to fetch it and got into his car. A huge feather blocked his view. It was in a bottle. He suddenly received a call. It was his teacher. She taught him to love. He searched for the file which she gave him. Then proposed her with a ring.

The story is very unrealistic to believe. Make your story as hilarious and unrealistic as possible so that it will stick for a longer time.

h) Songs

This method is easy for poems. Tune the poem into the tune of your favorite song and there you have it ready.

i) Movie

It is a technique which can be used for almost all subjects.
If it is history, visualize how the king ruled and waged a war.

If it is geography, visualize you going around all those places.
If it is chemistry, visualize how the chemicals interact with each other for the bonds to form.
If it is physics, visualize how the forces play with each other.
There is no limit to this technique. Leave the reins and let your creativity make the wildest movies which can stick for a lifetime.

j) Memory palace

It is similar to making a movie. But the location for the movie will be a known place, let us say your home. The characters will be moving around your room and using things which are available.

If you are studying about Indus valley civilization, the toys of that time are in your showcase. The jewelry of that civilization is in your living room.

k) Feel it

"I've learned that people will forget what you said, people will forget what you did, but people will never forget how you made them feel" - Maya Angelou.

Make use of emotions wherever you can to let it stick in your long-term memory.

l) Phone wallpaper

If you are looking for repeated reminder to remember a formula or concept, make it as your phone wallpaper of the day. Every time you unlock the phone, it reminds you of that. Don't keep it for more than a day because your mind would have already got used to it. If you want, you can repeat it after a while for spaced repetition.

7. Practice

a) Reading vs solving problems

I don't have time. Will going through how to solve the problems help me get through?

Does watching cricket matches day and night for 10 years make you a cricketer?

Does watching plays make you an actor?

Then how does seeing the solutions make you an expert at solving the problems?

If you want to avoid the same situation, solve the problems. Don't copy step by step. Try to do it on your own. If you can't do it, look at that part of the solution where you are stuck. Then try the remaining. Push yourself beyond what you are capable of. That makes your neurons struggle a bit more and strengthens them.

b) Take tests

When you write tests, it acts as a way of revision because you need to put in mental efforts to recollect.

Which tests are better?

When you answer a true or false question or a multiple-choice question, you happen to choose from one of them. You are not putting any efforts to recollect the answer. But if you must answer it in one sentence or write an essay on it, it helps in making you think about the topic in depth and helps in connecting it to other topics you know. This method facilitates chunking and connections too.

c) Teach the concepts

As a kid, my favorite game was to be a teacher. I could not afford to buy a board. I had a metal almirah at home which I used as the board. I explained my notes to imaginary students and wrote the key concepts on the transformed board. It was fun.

As I grew older, I always had a group of friends surrounding me before the exam to get their doubts cleared. If anyone ever called me on my landline at home, it was to get their doubts cleared.

Even though it is just a game to engage mind, it is one of the keyways to strengthen learning. You can acquire all the knowledge you require for the subject but what is the whole point if you can't retrieve or present it.

Teaching helps you achieve this. How to do this?

- You don't have to go in search of a student. You can do a mental image of how effectively you can present a topic
- If possible, help other students in your class. When I was in school, my teacher allotted a few students to me help them understand the concepts. That helped me to learn explain in layman terms
- If you can't find anyone to teach, you can write a blog or on question answer websites like Quora about what you understand about it. Using Quora for practicing my answers helped me in my presentation skills.
- Teach at an institute. After I stopped preparing for MBA entrance exams, I missed being in contact with the subject. I chose to be a teacher to help others achieve their dreams. I discovered techniques and understood concepts much better after I became a teacher.
- ☐

Chapter 9 - Distractions

After reading this chapter, you will learn

- What your distractions are
- How to avoid them
- How to concentrate

What are your distractions?

You tend to attend to everything other than academics. Your distorted selective attention causes distractions.

Now take some time and write down the list of your distractions.

What are your top 3 distractions of them?

1.
2.
3.

Which distractions do you think are causing the highest harms?

1.
2.
3.

Your top distraction may be a sound in the surrounding. Your mind might get diverted with the slightest sound you hear. But it does not do much harm because you immediately change your attention back to the subject. There is nothing much to dwell there. But if the distraction is a notification on your smartphone from a social media account, your life is screwed. It does not stop at the notification. You go deeper and check a few other updates. You go into the feed and browse through it endlessly.

In the end, when you are back to studies, your mind still lingers there. This is the distraction which causes the highest harm.

Common distractions

1.Noise in the background

In my school days, whenever I sat for studying, I used to hear noises of kids playing cricket on the ground floor of my building. Sometimes, it used to be first floor neighbors their TV volume too loud. Every single sound in the background used to bother me.

The most logical solution for this would be to listen to a music of your own in order to cancel out the background noise. But this has its own downsides.

- If the music has lyrics, your mind might be paying attention to the lyrics and not the subject you are studying
- Plain music also acts a sensory information which you need to ignore to divert your attention to the visual information
- You might get addicted to music and might not be able to study or write exams without it

The other solution for it would be to use earplugs to not let any sort of sound disturb you. But the dangerous side of this would be to not being able to hear sounds which are important like a fire alarm. Even though such occasions are rare, they are still a possibility.

You can also go to a library or a study center to minimize the number of sounds. Or make your room soundproof so that outside noises don't disturb you.

But the best solution, in this case, is to be interested in the subject, the details of which are in the ending of the chapter. This will help you concentrate anywhere and everywhere - classrooms, playground, exam halls. You can study anywhere with no trouble at all.

2. Social media

Using too much of social media affects your attention span. Your mind is distracted every time a notification pops up. As a result of which you can't focus on one thing beyond a minute. It also leads to multitasking where you not only stay on one app but jump to another before you get a reply on one. In the meantime, you browse through the app endlessly because you don't want to miss out on what is happening in everyone's life. While typing on the phone, you either use shortcuts or your phone autocorrects your spellings making you forget the basic grammar and spellings. The display light and the size of the letters hurt the retina.

At the end of all this process, you are not only distracted but also tired. Your mind only revolves around the endless updates you went through. You worry about the things not said. You fret over the things you said. In worst cases, you even go into depression for not being able to maintain a good profile online, virtual relations and a colorful and successful life to show off.

For example, let's see how WhatsApp alone can deteriorate your life.

a) Status

Once when I went to meet my friends, they were all busy checking status. What do you get by checking status? Maybe a dopamine rush of encountering something new. Another way to spend time? What is the reward in it?

b) Distraction due to Notifications

Every time you want to use your phone, there the messages are buzzing. Even after you disable the pop-up, you can see that a message has arrived. It is distracting all the time.

c) The expectation of a notification

When the expected notification does not reach you, you start getting irritated.

d) Group messages

Your phone is clogged all the time because the groups you are part of are buzzing with activity. Of what use is sending so many forwards all the time in all the groups which serve no purpose than wastage of time.

e) Decreased attention span

Working memory works the best when you concentrate on one thing at a time. When you send a text and expect a reply, your mind is on the text and not the work you do. Or even subconsciously you will be awaiting it.

f) Forgetting basic English grammar and spellings

Y does not have X's phone number.

The following conversation took place over WhatsApp.

X: "Can you send me your full name? They are asking for a background check."
Y: "Who are they?"
X: "IDK"

Y did not know what IDK stood for and thought it was the agency who was trying to do a background check.

g) Finger pain

One of my friends once complained that she was diagnosed with a finger pain due to over texting. Is WhatsApp worth the pain?

h) Psychological disorders

Excessive usage of WhatsApp can cause anything from irritability to bipolar disorder.

The best thing you can do for yourself is to come out of this trap.

- Keep your phone far away from your study place
- If you need it as a timer, switch off the connection to internet data or Wi-Fi
- If you must use it for referring to some information, change the settings in all the apps to no pop-up notifications
- Unless it is required for study purpose, delete all your accounts
- Turn off auto-correct suggestions
- Type as if you are writing an exam paper with right grammar and spellings.
- Don't get into virtual friendships. Go out and meet people in real
- Set a time aside in your day for using social media. Stick to your timelines strictly. Don't block your calendar for this neither in the morning nor in the night just before sleep. Also avoid it before intense study sessions.

3. Worry

Every second you spend in worrying can be used in learning a new concept. The more the time you worry, the greater the amount of the time you are losing.

Common worries of students

a) Syllabus

The syllabus looks scary when you have not attended the classes. Too many books covering the same material, is equally scary. The solution is simple. Don't look at it as a mountain to be climbed. Look at the small steps you need to take to finish it. Set small and reachable targets. Worry only about that. Not the entire syllabus. I was afraid of writing this book. I broke it into chunks. I started with writing 500 words a day for the first week. Then increased to 1000 a day for the next week. Then 1500 and finally 2000. If I looked at it as writing a book, I could have never written it.

b) Exams

"What if the question paper contains only the questions which I have not studied?"

"What if I forget everything by the time of exam?"

"What if the mind goes blank in the exam hall?"

The answer to the first question is covered in block 3. If you study according to the retention techniques mentioned in the last chapter, you don't have to worry about this. It is a problem only to crammers. Not everyone.

4.Love life

It is an unignorable part of life. Unless you are clear with your priorities clear and are aware of separating it from studies, it will haunt you throughout your student life.

a) You think about it all the time:

This takes you nowhere in life. It is like a dream with no goal. It takes a toll on your productivity. Instead, park it aside irrespective of your age. Every time a thought pops up, recollect a formula. It's simple. Just divert your mind.

b) You work for it all the time:

If that is what gives you what you want in life, set some time for it. Beyond that time, you are neither going to think about it nor act on it. This is easier said than done. The better option would be to postpone these plans till you reach your goal. The ultimate need for a human is to mate. But to mate and sustain a family you need to earn a living.

c) You are into it already:

This is easy. When I was in college, the class topper had a boyfriend. She perfectly managed studies and her love life. The secret was they were mature enough to dedicate a fixed amount of time for studies and for their love life. Another way this works in your favor is when both of you are into the same exam preparation, it helps in the subject discussion. In fact, this works best for you as all your needs are already taken care of. You need to focus on getting the bigger things in life. You can be glad that you are not in state one or two where you have to struggle for something. The only reason it works against you is when you are not into a mature relationship where you want to spend time with each other all the time.

d) Dealing with a breakup

One of my friends told me that she had a tough time to prepare for her exams because her boyfriend broke up with her just before exams. It is going to be tough. You are attached to someone for so long and when they withdraw it feels tough. You feel hopeless. That is the time you need to change your priorities in life.

Make your exam as the topmost priority. You might not get him back, but you can surely attract someone like him or better than him after the exam.

e) Make it work in your favor

When you are deeply infatuated with someone you will go to any length to impress them. Make that any length as studying. This will give you a good reason to top the exam. It is one of the easiest and best ways to stay motivated and achieve miraculous results. It doesn't matter if the person you want to impress changes with time; the better you score the better you stand at attracting the best.

5. Multitasking

I had the habit of listening to songs while doing homework. My mom used to come over and take my book off. She used to say "Enjoy the songs. You can study later." Those were the days when we did not have easy access to research papers on how multitasking will take you nowhere. Yet she disciplined me the right way.

In those days, it was songs or TV. But today you have a lot more distractions.

How to avoid multitasking?

a) Internet

When you are studying, you need just one website from which you are studying. Rest of the social media tabs are just for distraction. If you find it difficult to resist, don't save your password. You won't be that tempted to log in all the time.

b) Priorities

If you have 10 things to do for the day, don't do a little of one and then go for a little of the other. Order them on a priority basis of 1 to 10. Be realistic about how many can be achieved. Concentrate on them one after the other.

6. Thoughts

Keep a thought tracker. Whenever a thought pops up into your mind, make a note of it. If it is a serious one, you can work on it later. If it is a fantasy, you can become a writer and publish your stories. The reason why you should write it down is, once you release the thought on to the paper, you will reduce the rumination. Repeated thinking usually happens because your mind is afraid that it might forget it if you don't give the thought constant attention. Once you get rid of it, the working memory is freed up for your studies.

Other ways to tackle thoughts are

- Start reading the content loudly. This forces you to come back to reality
- Wear a stretchable wristband. Every time your mind wanders, hold it tight and release it. That little pain brings you back to the present.

7. Daydreaming

Even though this sounds like one of the biggest problems of students, it is a friendly distraction if you know how to turn it your advantage.

What did you daydream today? About being a superhero? Or did you daydream about sitting in a huge bungalow and living a comfortable life to not work for money again?

Whatever might be your dreams, keep dreaming (unless they are destructive).

But on one condition. Bring the subject you are studying into your dreams.
If you are studying organic chemistry, make the molecule sit along with you on the cushy sofa in your huge bungalow.

Molecule: "My name is Water."

You: "Hi Water. What is your molecular formula?"

Molecule: "H_2O. Why are you studying about me?"

You: "I need to know your properties. Can you tell me more about yourself?

Molecule: I have isotopes.........."

If you are studying history, imagine that you are interviewing the king. If that is not interesting enough, daydream about fighting a war with him.

Doing this has a lot of benefits for you

- You need not feel sad about not being able to concentrate
- You will remember better because of the fun involved in it
- Your creativity will improve

Downside to this:

Your situation will be better than the present but not the best. But to be the best you need to change the way you think and what you believe which is a long-term process. In the long term, you should improve your concentration, but for short term, you can try this.

How does this method work?

- Focused mode alone is not enough to remember what you read. You need your mind to relax and think about what you read in the backend. This is called diffused mode. We are converting your daydreaming mode to diffused mode of the brain.
- It is similar to memory palace/ association techniques
- Emotions help in pushing content to long-term memory. This fun will definitely help you remember better.

8.Sleep

Usually, you feel drowsy while studying either due to lack of proper sleep in the night or due to lack of nutritious food during the day. Even after fixing these both, if you are feeling drowsy, it means that you are not interested in the subject. There is no interaction happening between the short-term memory and the long-term memory.

Go back to the previous chapter and engage in active learning to avoid this state.

9.Addictions

I don't want to list the kind of addictions you might be prone to. If you don't have any addictions, you might develop one after knowing them. But whatever your addiction is, you need to understand the deeper reason underlying it. When you are addicted to something, it is not the object you are addicted to as you presume. It is the hidden feeling which you are trying to cover up under the name of addiction.

When a person is put in a healthy environment where he bonds with people around him in a natural way, he won't be addicted to one thing.

One of my friends told me that she keeps ordering food online once she is back home. She orders one after the other till she sleeps. As a result, she put on weight. She didn't order food because she was hungry. But ordered it because she was lonely. She didn't know if her stomach got full or not. But she needed food to keep herself happy. Is this any different from addiction? This girl was a social butterfly in college. Her room swarmed with friends all the time. Now when she has no one to connect with, she resorted to food.

If you are addicted to something

- Change your belief about it. Tell yourself that you don't need that to survive or overcome any feeling whatever you are using it for.
- Remove all the cues from the vicinity.
- Stay away from people who might be pulling you back into it.
- Find a healthier replacement. If you are addicted to chocolates, whenever you have a chocolate craving, have green tea instead.
- In the areas of your addictions, put a board of how important studying is for you.

General ways to avoid distractions

a) Time Tracking apps

You can use free apps like your time in your hand or rescue time. They will help you track where you are spending most of the time on your devices. This helps you to keep a limit on the same.

b) Rewards

For every study task you complete, bribe yourself with reward. Use this sparingly. Because intrinsic motivation helps in the long term than the external motivation.

The reward need not be something big. You can either use an app or make a chart and stick it in your room. You put a tick on the task once you finish it. I used loop tracker app and I find it rewarding enough.

c) Deadlines

Remind yourself of the deadline. I worked diligently on the book because I set a deadline for myself. I haven't finished the other books that I started writing because there are no deadlines for them.

d) Deep breathing

When your mind is wandering too much, a couple of deep breaths will be enough for you to come back to reality.

e) Pomodoro

Pomodoro is a time management technique where you study in intervals of 20-25 minutes. You don't have to worry about remaining focused for a long time. Remind yourself that it is just for this interval.

Download Pomodoro app. Do focused sessions.

f) Window

Don't sit beside the window. You are more prone to daydreaming every time you look out of the window.

Concentration

Is concentration a solution for your distractions?

It is often a misunderstood topic. Students think that concentration is a power. They need discipline and willpower to concentrate.

If you are also such a student, I have some good news for you. Concentration is not about willpower. It is about interest.

If your favorite movie or match is being telecasted on the TV, will you notice if a thief breaks into your house? Won't you be totally immersed? Because it is stimulating your mind.

When you are pursuing an activity, which is a little above your skill level and you find it a little challenging, you get into a flow state of mind.

So how do you concentrate?

Concentration is not about forcing yourself to study. Be interested in the topic. If you are not interested, cultivate interest by watching funny or interesting videos on the same topic.

Chapter 10 - How to study

After reading this chapter, you will learn

- Steps involved in studying
- Study groups
- Study areas
- Sample study plan

Getting into study mode

When you go to classes after a long break, you are physically present but mentally absent. Your focus is on everything but the class. You fight sleep while the lecturer stares at you.

This happens because

- The subject is too dry to sustain your attention
- There is no background story and direct information
- You don't find the topic interesting

What should you do?

1.Be interested in the subject:

Don't limit yourself to the course material. Watch some funny videos on it. Enroll for courses online. Buy fiction or nonfiction books on the subject. Do whatever it takes to get into the mode.

2. Accountability partner:

Make friends with people who are preparing for the same exam. Meet up. Talk about the subject. Share your struggles. Bond more. Discuss more.

Once you get into the mode, you will automatically start studying.

Planning the study

a) Time management

It is all about demand and supply. Everyone has the same 24 hours which is the supply. But demands are different for each person. If you increase your demands, the supply won't increase in any way. The only thing you can control is demands.

Let us see how you can manage your demands.

What are your demands for the day?

- Call friend
- Make notes
- Study today's syllabus
- Play with friends

Except for call friend, aren't rest of them part of the daily routine?

Time management now comes down to having a routine which has time for studying.

Routine for a school student

- School time
- Playtime
- Notes
- Tests
- Homework

Fill up your routines based on which category you belong to.

- School
- College
- Part-time employee
- Full-time employee
- Married full-time employee

After your routines are done, then you can talk about the other demands you have.

b) Timetable for the day

i) When should you plan it?

The previous day or the first thing in the morning

ii) What a typical list looks like

Subjects
Geography
History
Math

You mention the subject but not the topic. You will mention the topic but not what is the core concept you want to cover. Be specific.

What is the end goal you want to reach by visiting the concept? What questions can be asked in the exam from it? What can be the pitfalls? What is your key takeaway?

What your list should look like

Subject	Topic	Concept
Geography	Natural disasters	Earthquakes
History	Ancient Civilizations	Greek Civilization
Math	Geometry	Four-sided figures

Now don't stop there.
Allot the amount of time you are estimating it will take for it. The actual amount of time it takes to finish it might be more or less than this. You need not worry about it. But write down the time it takes.

Concept	Expected Time	Actual time
Earthquakes	1 hour	
Greek Civilization	2 hours	
Four-sided figures	3 hours	

Now allot an appointment with yourself for the day. In the time slot you assigned for yourself, you shall not do any other activity apart from meeting that subject.

Time of the day	Concept	Expected Time	Actual time
9 AM	Earthquakes	1 hour	
10 AM	Greek Civilization	2 hours	
2 PM	Four-sided figures	3 hours	

At the end of the day, go back to the schedule and mark what was the actual time you took to finish the concept. Mark the concepts which were not completed as incomplete and move them to another day's schedule. If you missed any time slot, write down your reason for it. With experience, you will be making a realistic schedule in the long run.

Time of the day	Concept	Expected Time	Actual time
9 AM	Earthquakes	1 hour	30 minutes
10 AM	Greek Civilization	2 hours	90 minutes
2 PM	Four-sided figures	3 hours	4 hours

Note:
One mistake which a lot of students make here is long study schedules with no time for eating and sleep. Remember that you are not a robot. Even robots need charging. You are a human. You need to rest in between. Keep your schedule realistic.
The second mistake is you force yourself to study all day with no entertainment. All work and no play makes Jack a dull boy.

c) When to take breaks?

Every person has a different concentration span. Figure out what is yours. This does not mean that you will just study for 5 minutes and call it as your concentration span. Fix the minimum as 20 minutes. Maximum of 1.5 to 2 hours. Even if you can concentrate beyond that there are chances that you will feel saturated. Take a 5-10 minutes break after each such session.

d) What to do in break time

1. Stretching exercises

Sitting at a place for a long time makes you feel tired. You will feel fresh and can also avoid back pain by doing some exercises in between.

2. Meditation

You have already dumped too much information into your brain. It needs some rest now. Meditation will help it consolidate the information.

3. Sky walk

When you study from a book, you bend your head for such a long time that the neck starts hurting. So walk for some time by looking at the sky. It relaxes your neck.

4. Walk

There are two types of thinking. One is focused work also known as convergent thinking. When you are studying, you are converging your thoughts. When you go for a walk, your brain moves into divergent thinking where it roams around. This helps your brain to form connections with the information you collected through convergent thinking.

5. Quick talk

You can indulge in a light talk which does not make you emotional or taxes your brain.

6. Laugh

Laughing helps you maintain the cheerful mode you require for the next study session. It will help you stay productive and creative. Go through comic books or watch some funny videos during the break time. In case you have wonderful friends, who can cheer you up and make you laugh, spend time with them. If you can't find any, try Hasyasana. It is a pose in yoga where you laugh for no reason. It helps.

e) What not to do in break time

1. Television

If you are a TV addict and watch TV during the break time, you will never be able to go back to studies. Even if you are back, your mind will be still stuck with TV.

2. Notifications

It does not stop with checking notifications. You will go through the endless feed. Then either get depressed or wonder why you must study when the entire world is not.

3. Long talks

If you get into an argument which has no end, there is no way you can get back to studies with a peaceful mind.

f) Which time of the day is effective for studying?

Power of morning hours

I am not asking you to wake up at 5 and study in Brahma muhurtham. In fact, there is a contradictory research that according to your Basic activity-rest cycle early morning 4 is the time when you are more likely to feel depressed.
So, it does not matter when you wake up, the best thing to do is make use of the fresh time for the most important dream of your life, which is studying.
Irrespective of how bad a mood with which you went for a sleep, in sleep, the toxic neurons die and you will be fresh in the morning.
Before you are bombarded with new problems or decisions in the day, use it to acquire the knowledge you want. Your mind is at peace and grasping power will be the highest.

You are a night owl. Should you still study in the morning?

There are controversial researches on whether you can study in the night or not. If you are drowsy all day and active in the night, that is the best time for you to study. There is no point in studying half-awake during the day when research asks you to study in the morning.

But studying in the night is usually counterproductive because your brain is already tired from the day. If you still want to go for nighttime studies, sleep after coming back from your daily routine of school or college or work. Then start with your studies because sleep helps in removing the tiredness.

If you are studying full-time at home, you can sleep in the afternoon too without feeling guilty as long as you keep up with the syllabus.

g) What to do while studying

1. Meditate before studying

My science teacher used to tell us to close our eyes before we start studying. I found that really helpful.

According to Hindu traditions, it is suggested to recite this Sanskrit sloka before we start studying.

Saraswati namasthubyam varade kamarupini
Vidyarambam karishyami bhavatumesada.

Greetings to Saraswati Goddess, the fulfiller of wishes. Please bless me in my endeavors towards studies.

You don't have to become a spiritual person for this now. But the below steps will help you get into studying mode.

Step 1:

Close your eyes. Breathe in. Breathe out. Repeat this ten times.

Step 2:

Make a note of all thoughts which disturbed you in the past few seconds on paper. Tell yourself that you are going to deal with them after your study time.

Step 3:

Tell yourself, "I am going to have a wonderful time studying. I enjoy learning new things. I am looking forward to them."

Step 4:

Recollect whatever you read previously if it is not a new topic.

Now you are ready to go.

2. Take a test before you start the subject

When you blindly study, you just retain whatever you find interesting. But when you take a test, you read with an end goal in the mind. You will have an idea of what you will be tested from the material. This further helps you pay more attention than what you do normally. You will end up scoring better in the tests.

Try this for yourself.

The policymakers of RBI did not change the price rates and maintained a neutral stance. This was quite predicted. Their primary remit has always been price stability. 4% of inflation is much above the medium-term target for a trend line. This gives us the clues to what might come up in the future. But it is never straight. The bimonthly monetary policy statement is confusing with no clear prediction as the way it looks at inflation and factors for price gains are different. The projections for CPI are lower than what it projected in the previous one.

The main factors mentioned by the RBI in reducing its inflation projections are a "sharp decline in vegetable prices and significant moderation in fuel group inflation." It anticipates the risks of deficit monsoon to food prices in spite of the forecast of a normal monsoon. Manufacturers are also expecting the prices to rise in their business. Volatility in oil prices was not given its due importance. Now GDP has become the main measure of economic growth instead of GVA. All this can confuse a common householder. They could have sent out clearer signals.

Question:

What factors does MPC take into account while changing the interest rates?

_____
_____
_____

How many factors are you able to write?

Now try this way.

What is the one point which the writer has been emphasizing throughout the para?

The policymakers of RBI did not change the price rates and maintained a neutral stance. This was quite predicted. Their primary remit has always been price stability. 4% of inflation is much above the medium-term target for a trend line. This gives us the clues to what might come up in the future. But it is never straight. The bi-monthly monetary policy statement is confusing with no clear prediction as the way it looks at inflation and factors for price gains are different. The projections for CPI are lower than what it projected in the previous one.

The main factors mentioned by the RBI in reducing its inflation projections are a "sharp decline in vegetable prices and significant moderation in fuel group inflation." It anticipates the risks of deficit monsoon to food prices inspite of the forecast of a normal monsoon. Manufacturers are also expecting the prices to rise in their business. Volatility in oil prices was not given its due importance. Now GDP has become the main measure of economic growth instead of GVA. All this can confuse a common householder. They could have sent out clearer signals.

Try to answer the question now.

What is the one point which the writer has been emphasizing throughout the para?

You will be able to answer it better because you know what you are looking for.

3. Speed reading

Start the timer here.

You should thank god for giving another beautiful day to live. You should thank god for giving you an opportunity to get ready freshly before the meeting. You should thank the traffic for diverting your mind from the pressure of the meeting and helping you relax for some more time. All these sounds counter-intuitive and look like excuses. But I call it as looking for the good in the bad.

I embarked on a 30-day positive challenge and fell sick for a week. I had no other choice than to thank god that whatever my illness was, it was curable. I am thankful to have parents who took care of me when I was sick. I am thankful to have a job where I will not be removed from the rolls for taking off for a week. I am thankful to have colleagues who worked over-time to do my share of work.

But excuse me, my friend, this is not a change which comes overnight. You need a shift in thinking. If you think that way today and go back to what you are tomorrow, it is not going to help. You need to look for the positive in the negative in every thought. This is going to be tough. But definitely doable.

Start doing this small exercise today. Daily write one thing you are grateful for. Every night before you go to sleep, write this. Tell me the change you see in a month.

Stop the timer.

Divide 249 by the number of minutes you took.
That gives your words per minute.

Again start the timer.

You had a great start to the year with lofty resolutions. 15 days into it, you feel lost. You can't find your path. You feel like a loser. You want to change for the better. You want more out of your life. But nothing seems to be working. You are drowned till your neck in your work with zero work-life balance.

Hold on for a second. Take a deep breath. Breath in breath out. Now read further.

Everyone has 24 hours a day. Some people achieve more while some people achieve less at the same time.

How can you fall into the achieve more category?

Even though these are clichés, I want to still repeat them.

Do

1.Sleep well

It is not about the number of hours you sleep but how deep your sleep was. Wake up naturally and not for an alarm. Feel fresh when you wake up so that you don't feel sleepy throughout the day.

2.Exercise

It increases your stamina. You won't come back home and complain that you had a long day. It gives you enough energy to play with your children after a tiring day at the office.

3. Eat Breakfast

When your stomach keeps growling, there is no way you can focus on work. Your brain will be more active when you feed it with the right amount of food on time.

Don't

4. Keep checking notifications

Whenever I was free, I used to open WhatsApp and Gmail to check for notifications. After a point of time, I was so fed up with myself that I removed those apps from my home screen. Now I placed kindle app on home screen, and I will read a page of a book in my break time.
There is no end to notifications and feed on social media. It is going to eat up your time endlessly.

Now that you got your basics right, this technique will work for you.

5. Make an IF …. THEN list

According to this list, you are going to use the free time which you created by getting rid of your social media notifications.

This is my list.

1. If I am waiting for a cab, then I will speak one line in Tamil with my colleague
2. If I am waiting in a queue, I will read a book
3. If I want to listen to songs, I will do a course instead
4. If I want to text out of boredom, I will write on Quora.

The above list might look insignificant.

If I talk for even 240 days in Tamil, I will become good at basic Tamil.
If I read even one page a day, I can finish a book in a year.

If I listen to 5 minutes of a course a day, I will finish a course in a month.
If I write one answer a day, I will have 365 answers in a year.

Stop the timer.

Divide 513 with the number of minutes it took for you.

This gives your words per minute.
For a lot of students, the second one takes lesser time than the first one. The reason being simple. The second text is more organized, and you know what to expect when you read it. So it helps in faster reading.

When you read a dry text which is in the form of continuous paragraphs, you have to either imagine it all as you read or summarize the para in one word in your head to help in quick retrieval.

You can go do techniques of speed reading but the amount of efforts you put in speed reading if you put in learning the concepts, it will help you achieve success quicker.

To summarize

- For text with continuous paragraphs, you need to make notes
- For text which is already in an organized way, you already read fast

So, don't worry about speed reading.

4.What to do after reading?

- Write the summary of the entire page in a few words. If you just read those words, it should summarize the entire page
- You can make mind-maps if the number of concepts is a lot
- Draw a funny picture if possible

- Use the techniques from retention chapter to make the reading stick

Now it is time to test whether you remember what you read or not.

5. Mock tests

Write as many tests as possible before the actual test.

When I was in school, my mom used to set a mock paper for me. I had to write it like an exam, and she used to correct it. It served a dual purpose of recollecting instead of rereading. I also got to know my areas for improvement and the mistakes I was prone to make.

As I grew a little older, since it was not possible to write it all before the day of the exam, she used to make me answer all the questions and correct me where I recited wrong points or the ones which I did not know well.

When it came to my preparation for entrance to engineering colleges, I joined an institute which made me write a mock test every week. It was rigorous but I got feedback on a regular basis on my strengths and weaknesses. I knew where I stood at class, city, state and country level.
When I prepared for MBA entrance exams too, I made sure that I enrolled for mock exams which gave a detailed analysis on my strong and weak areas and difficulty level of questions I was answering.

At every stage of my life, I would have never achieved what I did without the numerous mock tests I took. Taking multiple tests makes the final test just another test. You will no longer fear it because it is just another test in the list of tests.

Why should you take a mock test?

- You will know your strong and weak areas.

- It will give you a feel of the actual test environment
- It will help you overcome test anxiety
- It is a better way of revision than re-reading
- If it is an external test it will give you a rough idea of the competition you need to face
- Improves your attention
- Reduces test fear
- It will help you build a strategy for the test

When should you take a mock test?

First mock test

You should take the first mock test before you start your preparation. It gives you an idea of where you stand with no preparation. If you can't answer a single thing on the paper, don't freak out. If you are able to answer a lot of them, don't feel overwhelmed. Analyse the paper with a balanced mind and chalk out your preparation based on that. If you have an opportunity, analyze it with an expert or mentor who will guide you on how to make a preparation plan based on that.

Next mock tests

As you keep progressing with your basics, take subject-wise mock tests. This helps you gauge your understanding of the topics. The syllabus looks less intimidating. If you don't do well in any of the tests, it gives you a chance to revisit the basics before it is too late. At this stage, you can take occasional full-length mock tests based on your comfort, confidence levels and time availability.

Time of the day

This plays a major role in tuning you to tests. Take tests in all sorts of scenarios. Write tests when you are fresh in the morning, back from a heavy dinner, when you are dead tired after class or work, when you are sick and can't even get up from the bed.

Even though the above seems like the weirdest advice you ever received, for my school level exam, I had severe cramps and could not bear the pain in the mid of exam. All I wanted to do was run away from the exam hall. During my class 12 final exams, I had a sprain in my back and could not move my neck. It was a torture. I had to write my engineering entrance test after taking an IV injection which induced drowsiness and constrained my hand movement. I had no strength to even sit for the exam but managed it with glucose water. You never know what might happen a day before an exam or on the day of the exam or in the exam hall.

Environment

Take tests in all types of environment. Write them in a calm and peaceful environment, when your sibling is watching your favorite show on TV when your friend is indulging in your favorite gossip, when the song you hate the most is being played in the background.

When I wrote one of my engineering entrance exams, the invigilators were talking loudly. I found it irritating and found it tough to focus on the exam. It might sound stupid but it prepares you for the worst.

How should you take a mock test?

1.Online/Offline

If your exam is going to be online, take as many online tests as possible. A few students have trouble looking at the screen for long hours. You will know if you also have any such issues. You can either go for getting corrective glasses or eye liquid to prevent drying your eyes.

For an offline preparation, it is easy to underline and highlight. It won't be the same for online. So, if it is an online exam, practice the tests online.

Also, for solving problems, you must look at the screen and the paper, it is a distribution of attention between the screen and the paper.

For offline exams, if it involves marking the OMR sheet, practice on the same type of paper. I made a mistake in marking the hall ticket number on the OMR sheet for one of my engineering entrance exams because the 0 was at the front in my mock papers and it was at the last in the main exam paper. When your brain is trained to do something, you will automatically make a few mistakes.

If it is a subjective paper, practice writing neatly. For a second, think you are the examiner. If you have to read bundles of papers to evaluate them, will it give you a pleasant feeling to read illegible handwriting?

He won't be spending more than 5 minutes in reading your paper. Will he be willing to read to comprehend the long illegible essays in detail to give you full marks?

Rules for writing well

- Write neatly
- Underline the important points
- Draw flowcharts and tables wherever possible
- Don't strike too much. In case you do, do it as a single strike instead of making it look like a block

2. Environment

In the present generation, one of the biggest problems students face is attention span. They are constantly bombarded with notifications from different social media and are totally into multitasking. You might feel close to impossible to sit a place at a stretch and write without talking or accessing other websites.

When you write mock exams, the first thing you are trying to work on is concentrating for that long without any distractions. The challenge in the first mock will be to sit for 2 hours or 3 hours at a stretch. The more tests you take the concentration part will be taken care of.

3. Timings

Even though in the previous section I mentioned that you should write in all possible times, as the exam time approaches start writing exams during the time slot of the actual exam. This helps you set your biological clock in sync with the exam. You also will start waking up and eating at the same time as you will be doing on the actual day of the exam.

4. Frequency

After 60% of the basic syllabus is done, you can start taking full-length mock tests a bit more regularly than before. As you reach 80% of the syllabus you can write one in a week.
After the syllabus is completely done you can write two or three a week. But in a week before the exam, limit the number of tests you write

5. Brand

Choose the mock tests which give you

a) Detailed analysis

Irrespective of whatever details they give, you will have to work a bit more to customize it to your level. But it will be helpful to get the basic level analysis.

b) City, State, country ranks

Even though it does not predict your actual rank, it will give you a rough idea of where you stand

c) Variety of questions

A question paper should not be a standard set or type of questions. It should have a mix of everything. If it is too predictable, it might not serve the end purpose.

d) Different levels of question papers

The level of the set of mocks you take should not be the same level. It should be a mixture of easy, medium and difficult. The same is backed by an experiment on 8-year-olds where they had to toss bean bags into buckets which are 3 m away. One set practiced only 3m away and other set practiced 2m and 4m away. In the final exam, the latter set scored better than the first set.

What should you do after a mock test?

If you are not doing this step, the use of taking a mock test is useless.

Writing a mock is just a part of the process. Analyzing it makes the difference.

Why should you analyze?

- It tells your strong and weak areas
- It tells you the efforts you need to put in to get the desired score

- It tells you the factors due to which you are not able to do well
- It tells you the areas where you have to go back and read

How should you analyze?

First look at the overall score. Is it close to what you expected? If it is not, it means that you have marked too many answers wrong. It could be either due to

- Silly mistakes
- Wrong understanding of the subject
- Too many guesses

Is it close to what you desired?

If it is not, you must work on the mistakes you have made in this test to reach the desired mark in the next test.

What are the types of mistakes you are making?

- Not reading the question properly
- Missing the key word in the question
- Lack of subject knowledge
- Calculation mistakes
- Stuck between two options
- Marking the wrong answer even after knowing the right one

Now classify your wrong answers and unanswered questions under these mistakes. If you made any other type of mistake write them too.

Now work on each of them individually. You will learn in detail on how to do well in exams in the next block.

When should you analyze?

Research shows that analyzing immediately is not as helpful as analyzing it after a while. But don't delay it for too long that you have forgotten about the test completely.

How to learn more from tests?

Most of the times you will only look at the rightly or wrongly marked answer option. But when the test setter composes the test paper, he won't do inky pinky ponky to set the question and answer options. A bit of logic and thought process goes into it. Let's take this question for example.

Is the following statement true?

Private bill can be proposed by a member of parliament and the President holds final decision to approve or reject it.

If you don't know about this question, identify the keywords and learn about them.
What is a private bill?
Who is a member of parliament?
When is a private bill produced?
What are the criteria to be a member of parliament and what are his duties?
What are the duties and entitlements of the president of India?

If you already know the answers for them, quickly recollect them. In the actual test, something similar to this might occur. Use every part of the question for revision.

What to do when you are stuck in a problem or concept?

The other day in my class, a student was not solving problems. I was concerned. I asked him "Why are you not solving any problems?" He replied, "I don't understand anything!"
He was lying. So are you.
You know the language you are reading the problem in. You will understand something but not everything.

Follow a step by step approach to finding the root cause

Step 1: List down the problem areas. Which parts of the problem are you not able to understand?

Step 2: Why are you not able to understand? Is it lack of subject knowledge or confusion?

Step 3: Select one problem area to start with.

Step 4: Narrow down the problem further. Define the problem clearly.

Step 5: What are the resources required to fix it? Will asking a friend or teacher help? Or is that knowledge you require is available in any material?

Step 6: Apply it and fix the problem.

Step 7: Repeat the same for other problem areas too.

Step 8: Combine all the solutions and your problem is solved.

By using this approach, you will be able to do root cause analysis for your obstacles in problem-solving. This in turn helps you go a long way in approaching new types of problems in exams.

6. Study groups

When to form one?

Don't form a study group for learning the concepts. You can't have a common timetable because each of you has a different grasping capacity.

Form the group when you are thorough with what you have studied and want to teach the concepts to others or to get other's perspective.

Why form one?

It is not compulsory to have a study group. But it is useful in the following cases

- When you need a different perspective
- When you are not able to generate enough points
- When you are confining yourself to home and need to socialize
- When you were not able to understand a few concepts by yourself

How to select one?

a) Same level

Once when I was in engineering, I found it impossible to study with a friend. She looks at the slide and immediately grasps it. I needed some time to understand the details of it. If you can't grasp or understand at the same speed, one of them for sure is going to get frustrated quickly.

b) Same type

With another friend, I used to find it difficult to study together because she just crams it all. I need to take time to understand and make notes. I can't memorize without a background on the topic.

c) Complement each other

You are strong in a few areas and your study mate in a few other areas. Both of you can help each other.

How to sustain one?

- Contribute to the group
- Meet at regular intervals
- Don't gossip

7. Study area

All through my school days, my mother had a tough time arranging my books. I used to spread them all over the table and study. Needless to mention about the rough papers. She never understood which ones to keep and which ones to throw away. It was a total mess.

How should you keep your study area?

1. Table/chair

Do you have a dedicated study table? If yes, don't fill it with books. Keep the ones which you are referring to now. If you keep the books which you are going to read for the entire day it will only cause you anxiety.

If you don't have a study table and low on budget, you don't have to worry. You can get a chair and a plank along with it to sit in a comfortable posture. If you don't even want to spend on that you can always use the dining table.

If there is nothing available, you can sit cross-legged on the floor. My father used to make me sit this way and study. It is a yoga posture which is known to calm the body and relax it.

2. Arrange your books

Arrange the books either by the subject or group them based on notebooks, textbooks or reference books. Choose the way you can remember well. Get a marker and write along the side what each subject is so that you can identify them easily. There is no fun in searching through the entire dump for the book you need. You will end up wasting all the energy you need for studying in searching for the book.

3.Papers/Notebooks

If you are doing rough calculations which you don't have to refer to again, you can use loose papers. Trash them once the job is done.

In case you want to write notes, it is always better to get a notebook. Maintain an index for it. Mention the date and the topic which you are studying. This helps in searching for the points you made on the topic easily at a later point in time.

4.Sitting posture

Sit straight. If you are studying in a sleeping posture, there is no point in complaining that books make you sleep. If you are resting your face on your palms, that will also make you take a nap. Sit in a way which is conducive to studying.

5.Lighting

Eyes feel good when you study in a naturally ventilated room. Don't let any shadow fall on your book when you are studying or writing. If you are studying during the night time, choose only well-lit rooms.

6.Clothes

In tropical countries, not everyone can afford an air-conditioned room for studying. If you have to sit for long hours for studying in summer make sure that you are wearing loose cotton clothes. They not only enable a free flow of air but also help in better absorption of sweat. If it is winter, don't use a blanket to keep yourself warm. It is a sure shot way of going to sleep. Wear thick clothes and sweater to keep yourself warm.

7.Posters

Your eyes notice only what is different from before. So motivational posters don't really help in the long term. If you want the posters to work for you, you need to keep changing them. They will also help you when you lack motivation and need some encouraging words.

8.Do not disturb board

When I was in a hostel, I wrote this on the door when I did not want to be disturbed while studying. Unless you have sadistic people around you, it is quite often helpful.

9.Designated areas

Should you stick to only one place as your study area?

Having a designated study area helps you get into study mode as soon as you enter into it. But if you are already in a study mode/mood, vary your areas. This acts as a retention technique because along with the content you will associate the area too. It helped me a lot.

Libraries

1. Existence/Availability

Will it affect your studies if you don't have access to a library?

All through my school days, I found the library a blessing in my life. It was an age where the internet was not rampant and cheap. For all sorts of information, I needed to rush to a library. But today having access to a library is not as important as it was a few years ago. Do a quick search on the net if you have access to one. If you don't have one, you don't really have to worry about it. You can find other ways to get access to the same. But if you are still a college student, you always have the advantage of having a college library.

2. Paid/Free

Issues with free libraries:

The library which was a few meters away from my house was always crowded. If I had to get a decent place to sit, I have to go the library the first thing in the morning. The book I want to read might also have been already taken away by someone. There will be too many people fighting for too little resources.

But the advantage of this is it will provide you motivation to study harder.

Is it worth paying for a library?

If the library is going to provide you colorful books which will accelerate your learning, you can go ahead and pay for it. Another reason why a lot of students need a library is for peaceful, no disturbance environment for studying. These days you have air-conditioned study centers which provide you the same environment. You can rent them per month.

3. Read at library

Environment

One of the best things the library provides in this age is the environment to study without any disturbances. Psychologically, you tend to do better when you are a part of an environment which does the same. So this environment is conducive to you.

You might find an accountability partner. Even if you don't feel the motivation on the first day, you will feel accountable to go to the library to study.

Note making

If you are going for referring the books, don't make an entire copy of the book. Refer to the note making section to read more on how to make notes.

Borrow books

I prefer borrowing books than buying books. When I buy a book, I feel that the book is going to be there forever. What is the hurry to study it today? When you borrow a book, it comes with a return date. You will feel pressured to finish the book before the return date.

Do they still play a role in the digital age?

If you want a library for the sake of referring to some additional information, you have google books or research papers online. You don't have to take the pain to go all the way to a library.

How to use a library to succeed in an exam?

- Use it for a study environment
- Write mock tests
- Find an accountability partner

How does library deter you from succeeding in an exam?

- Spending too much time to reach the library
- Making friends who kill your time
- Referring to too many books and forgetting the bigger picture

8. Internet

- Helpful in watching videos related to the subject.
- A few websites would have already created the necessary mind maps
- Free or paid online tests

Things to remember

Source:

Not all sources are reliable. Everyone out there is busy churning out content. It is important to know if they get their data from reliable sources

Distraction:

When I want to do research on something, I end up having more than one tab open. This leads to multi-tasking which in turn affects my studying

9. Reference Books

Should I study from reference books too?

- If you don't have much time for exams, don't spend time reading extra books
- If you have a lot of time before exams, reading reference books helps you develop an interest in the topic and also gives you the context for the dry academic textbooks

10. New textbooks

Should I buy new textbooks every year?

- If the exam paper pattern changes every year, the newer books will have the latest information
- If the facts are going to be updated every year, it is better to have the latest edition
- If you have a dust allergy, avoid the old books

11. How to deal with the fear of failing during preparation?

You overcome the fear of failure by embracing it.

Fail today in solving the problems and not in the exam. It will hurt in the beginning that you are far behind your counterparts. You feel all the efforts going waste. But wait! Was it a waste? Your mind needs a bit of struggle to remember well. That is the state you are in. When you do the next round of preparation you know that it was all a way to make you remember more effectively.

If you really failed in solving a problem, you know what methods don't work. The one who succeeded only knows one way. The way to get the problem right. If you tweak the problem a little, he will be confused. He will start fearing failure.

But since you failed to solve the problem, you know of all the ways which don't work. A tweaked problem in the exam won't scare you. After all the failures you will succeed with top marks in the exam.

After failing to solve a problem or understand a concept, you know the exhaustive ways in which things don't work. You are more knowledgeable.

The one who succeeded would have done by chance. His knowledge is limited to only one way of getting the answer right. He doesn't know the obvious ways in which one can make mistakes.

So, fail today. Embrace the feeling. Learn from the experience. And fail in a greater way tomorrow. Make all the mistakes in the preparation stage.

Failure does not define what you are as a person. It does not mean anything at all.

Who is called a failure?

The one who has failed according to the dictionary definition and considered himself a failure.

If you stop studying because you feel like a failure, that is when you are called a failure.

What can you do to stop feeling this?

Reward yourself for the efforts and not for the result.

Question yourself every day – Am I enjoying this?

12. Sample study plan

Let's say your exams are going to start in 45 days. You have 6 subjects. It is a subjective exam for which you don't want to cram the subject at the last minute.

Your first step is to search for mock exams or previous year question papers. You can search for this either on the university page or other websites which would have posted the same. If you don't want to use the internet to avoid multitasking, you can purchase a book for the same. This will give you an idea of what the question paper will be like. You will know the way you have to retrieve the content in the exam hall.

The next step is to deal with the syllabus. What is your studying speed? How do you want to chunk it for 45 days? Since the days are fixed, you have to make more time during the day to accommodate the syllabus. If you had more time, you could have reduced the amount of time spent on each day in studying.

Since you have very short time left, you can read only from your textbooks. Each subject has 16 chapters. When you have to count for all the 6 subjects, you need to study 96 chapters. If each chapter takes one hour, you need 96 hours for studying. Since you might want to have a few cheat days in between, you need to spend 3 hours daily on studying to finish it in 32 days.

Since you are going into a study mode after a long time, you will give up easily if you start with 3 hours a day. You can start with one hour a day per week. This can be easily accommodated in the evening. Later slowly increase it to 2 hours a day per week. You can wake up a bit earlier and accommodate one more hour. In the third week, you can split it to one and half hours in the morning and one and a half in the evening. In the fourth week, you can pull 10 minutes here and there during the day and study for half an hour more.

Week 1 - 1*7 = 7 hours
Week 2 - 2*7= 14 hours
Week 3- 3*7= 21 hours
Week 4 - 3.5*7= 24.5 hours
Week 5 - 4*7 = 28 hours

This will roughly cover the entire syllabus in 5 weeks without feeling stressed out.

You can read a chapter from the different subject every day. So that you can repeat the subject after 6 days in the first week. After that, you can repeat them in 3 days and so on.

In between, you can write a few mock tests to test yourself and also to strengthen the retention. After that, you can go back and use a few more previous year question papers as mock tests and practice what you learned.

Block 3-Exam strategy

Studying is just one part. Scoring well on a test is a totally different ball game. You might be the most knowledgeable person in the class but if you can't write the exam well, you will never be able to get what you always wanted.

It happened with me. I was preparing for CAT, the entrance examination for MBA colleges in India. I had all the subject knowledge. Even if you wake me up in the middle of the night, I can solve any question for you. But when it came to the exam, my mind used to go blank. It happened every year and I lost hopes of ever getting through it.

I decided to write this book so that I can help many others who are knowledgeable and are still not able to get through due to various reasons.

Chapter 11 - What to expect in the exam

After reading this chapter, you will learn

- How to set your mind for the exam

When you are preparing for the exam, you find a few concepts effortless to remember. You wish the examiner tests you on those. But in the examination hall, when you see the questions are on the concepts which you are not confident, you get a mild shock. This in turn disturbs the mind and makes retrieval tough. Instead, if you prepare your mind for the exam, irrespective of the level of the question paper, you will still do well.

How to know what to expect?

1.Previous exam papers

If you ever want to excel in an exam, you should not undermine the importance of going through the past exam papers. Not because the same questions might be repeated but it will help you predict what the future papers will be like.

If you want to top the exam, it will tell you what topics you should never leave. If you want to pass the exam, it will tell you what topics alone you can study and still pass.

School

When I was in school, I used to go to the library either during lunch or after school to go through the exam papers. Just before the day of the exam, I used to get calls from my friends asking for important questions. I could predict the questions correctly 80% of the time. Not because the paper setters were fools but you can get the throb of the paper setter by looking at the question paper.

My predicting skills got so well with time that I daringly prepared for only 5 essays in Hindi subject for my 10th class boards. 3 of the 5 I prepared for appeared in the exam.

Even today, when one of my friends expressed her fear that her daughter might fail in Tamil paper, I asked her to visit the library and have a look at previous question papers and train her daughter on the topics which have low cost and high benefits. No prizes for guessing. Her daughter passed with little efforts.

University level
A professor has a lot more work to do than setting a novel question paper every year. The questions can either be a twist on the previous year or if you are lucky enough to get hold of papers of a lot of years, you might even get the same question you practiced before.

Objective competitive exams
If the exams can be taken at any time in the year, the level of paper will be more or less the same. By following a standard test series, you will be able to gauge the level of exam and type of questions to expect.
If the exams are conducted once or twice a year, a look at the previous question papers tells you whether they maintain the same level or have a different surprise element every year. Either way, you are prepared for it.

Subjective competitive exams

If the exam is based on the same syllabus, you can predict the important topics which they usually test on. If it is based on current affairs, you can expect a surprise.

In short, if the exam is a type of exam which is known for surprises, be ready for it. If it is a predictable one, make sure that you are familiar with the predictable parts.

2. Classes
If you pay attention in classes, teachers tell you what to expect in the exam and how to approach it. If you make note of it as and when they tell you, it will come handy at the last minute.

3.Mock exams
When you start writing exams, you will understand how to approach the paper.

Chapter 12-Before the exam

After reading this chapter, you will learn

- What to do at various lengths of time before the exam
- How to deal with exam stress and other unexpected events

Planning for exams

What to do a year before the exam?

Write one mock exam. It tells you where you stand. You will know what your current ability level is. To reach your desired level, you will know how much effort you need to invest.

Analyse the paper,

- How many questions did you answer?
- How many of them did you answer confidently?
- How many did you guess?
- What was the difficulty level of the ones you answered - easy or tough?
- What were your pain points while solving the paper?
- Were the questions you answered were all from the same topic or different topics?
- What was your confidence level?

After you are done analyzing the above, you will know what your strong and weak areas are. You will know what to expect from the paper and what to expect from yourself.

Now for the next 6 months focus on the basics.

Refer to the chapter on acquiring subject knowledge. During this time, write subject wise tests to check yourself periodically. Once in two months, you can write a full level test too. Once you are thorough with the basics, start writing tests once a week. That is the best way to practice and also to revise the concepts.

What to do 6 months before the exams?

You won't have the luxury to spend much time on concepts. Try to finish them in 2 months and concentrate on sharpening your basics by writing exams after that.

What to do 3 months before the exams?

You can still follow the 6 months strategy, but you will have less time to master your exam strategy.

At this point, I want to address an important issue. 2 months might not be realistically possible for a few students to start learning the concepts from basics. If you think you need more time, for a competitive exam you can write the main exam with whatever knowledge you have by then, only if the attempt does not cost you much.

What to do a week before the exam?

- Watch out the food you eat. Don't eat any outside food or heavy oily food. Eat a fruit a day.
- Get proper sleep.
- Align your sleep and food cycle based on your exam timings.
- Stop worrying about what you didn't cover.
- Spend time in meditating and staying calm.
- Recollect whatever you have studied.
- Don't reread the entire syllabus

What to do the day before the exam?

- Let the mind be in a diverged state. It is the state of mind where you don't do work and where you need to focus your thoughts. Feel free.
- Visualize how you are going to avoid the regular mistakes. If you are someone who does frequent calculation mistakes, visualize that you write the numbers correctly and then recheck them.
- Check clearly what subject exam you have the next day - Once, one of my friends prepared for a subject different from the actual subject for the exam. Don't make that mistake.
- Prepare a checklist of items you need to carry to the exam hall. Usually, list contains
    - Pens
    - Pencils
    - Geometry box
    - Water bottle
    - Chewing gum or chocolates (if allowed)
    - Hall ticket
    - Wristwatch
    - Calculator (Make sure the battery is full)
- Decide what you are going to wear. Dressing affects your mood significantly. Wear something you love and feel comfortable in
- Check the exam center the day before. Going to the wrong exam center will cost you a lot

What not to do the day before the exam?

- Learn or cram anything new
- Tax yourself emotionally
- Write mock tests
- Worry about the topics you didn't study
- Call friends and inquire about how they are feeling

What to do the night before the exam?

- Most importantly get good sleep.
- Stop getting into discussions and avoid all sorts of screens an hour before your sleep time.
- Eat something healthy and not too heavy. Finish dinner by 8.
- Don't fret. Revise something light if you think you need to. But avoid rereading. Try to recollect the flowcharts or the key points which you are afraid that you might forget. But again, don't fret if you can't recollect. It is all there in your mind. Refer to your notes to strengthen a concept which you can't recollect.

If you have difficulty falling asleep

- Try deep breathing. Tell yourself repeatedly that you are going to perform well in the exam
- If that does not work, listen to music which induces sleep.
- If you are still disturbed by thoughts, take a note pad and make a note of the thoughts. Tell yourself that you are going to deal with them after the exam.
- Even though it is not recommended, if you are an insomniac, you can see a doctor and get tablets for the sake of exams. You don't want the long duration preparation efforts to go down the drain because you could not get a proper sleep the night before.

Pre-Exam Stress

1.You haven't studied anything

Since you read the book till here, you don't belong to this category. But if you are looking for some shortcuts, you need to relax. Irrespective of whether you are tensed or not tensed, the chances of you passing the exam are low. But if you are calm, there is at least a little chance of passing.

If it is a subjective exam, you need to know at least a few keywords. If the question asks you to write about human heart you should at least know where it is located and what its function is to show that you at least know something if not for the details.

If it is an objective exam with no negative marking, since you anyway don't know anything, there is no harm in going through the paper to look for questions which can be answered by common sense. There will be at least a few for which you don't really have to possess subject knowledge, yet you can answer them. Exhaust those questions first. Later, choose one option and select the same for all of them. When you toss a coin, the probability of head or tail is 50% when it is done on a mass scale. Similarly, if there are a hundred questions, the probability of any option is the number of questions divided by the number of options. If the paper is set by a human, there are higher chances for the option to be the middle ones. For example, if there are 100 questions and the answer options are A, B, C, D then the chance of any option being right is close to 25% and either B or C might have the higher probability to be right. You can just test your luck.

2.You have studied a few topics only selectively

When you study selectively, you will have the fear of questions appearing only from the syllabus which you have not covered. Even in this case, there is no point in worrying. While selecting the topics itself, be careful about the topics you select. Do your selection based on the pattern of previous question papers. Take a calculated risk. The most important thing is to not get tensed if there are a very few questions from the topic you selected. Forget that the remaining questions exist on the question paper and answer what you know.

3. You left a few topics only selectively

At this stage don't expect to top the test. There might be a few questions which might come from the topics you did not cover. But keeping your mind cool will help you give your best in what you already know.

4. You studied everything

Worry of these types of students is of two types

- Recollecting the content during the exam
- Worrying about getting a question out of the syllabus

The first worry can be fixed by studying with methods mentioned in the book which help in longer retention. The second worry is imaginary. The sooner you realize the better.

Dealing with anxiety

Own it up.

You can't feel better unless you want to feel better. Tell yourself that you are feeling anxious and that it is perfectly okay. You are human and there is nothing wrong with that feeling. Even though anxiety remains after doing this, it is easier to take action after acknowledging. If you don't know what the problem is, how will you ever solve it?
If the stress or anxiety is severe, conditions like continuous yawning due to anxiety, shivering hands and legs, stomach upset and nausea, see a psychologist before the exam to deal with that.

Dealing with low performance

Even though mocks help you understand where you stand, they are not the end of life. I have seen many students and also friends who did terribly in mocks but came out with flying colors in exams.

One of my friends who barely got 36 percentile in mocks, scored 91 percentile in the main exam.

The main exam was much easier than the mock test and she did the right question selection technique and she performed well.

So don't let them define you.

Depression

First, understand that it is common to feel depressed during the long duration of exam preparation. You are bound to feel hopeless and restless.

What to do when you feel that?

- Take a deep breath. Exhale out the pessimism and inhale the optimism. Imagine the negativity going out through the nostrils and the positivity walking in through the nostrils.
- Go through your past achievements. If you are feeling low about the future, go through the good times of the past. Whenever you think you did well about something, appreciate yourself for it. Make a note of it. This list comes handy during the depressing times.

- Do something you love. Don't force yourself to study more when you are depressed. Take a break. Pamper yourself. Feel loved. Come back and study.
- Don't talk to people about how doomed you are. It is important to overcome the feeling that whatever you have studied is a waste and you will never be able to make it. The more you talk about it, the more you feel it. So, stop talking about that and distract yourself from the feeling. As long as you are true to your efforts, you don't have to worry about the end result.

Fear of failure

A few students skip taking the exams because they are afraid of failing to reach up to expectations. By succeeding in life, you have escaped an event where you didn't fail. But for how long will you escape? Every day you have to live in the fear 'What if I fail tomorrow?!'. You will limit yourself to only those ways where you know how to succeed. Don't you want to explore and reach new heights?

If you don't write the exam tomorrow, you will have a regret of "I should have tried." Life of regrets is worse than a life of efforts not yielding the best result. When you have all the chances to get your desired result, you are ruining every chance of success by contemplating the failure of it.

How to overcome the fear of failure?

Don't focus on the result.

You did everything possible to achieve the best result for tomorrow's exam.

The result is not in your control. Trying to control anything which is not under our control always leads to stress. This stress further deteriorates your health and state of mind which ruins your chances of succeeding.

karmaṇy-evādhikāras te mā phaleṣhu kadāchana

mā karma-phala-hetur bhūr mā te saṅgo 'stvakarmaṇi

Translation: You have a right to perform your prescribed duties, but you are not entitled to the fruits of your actions. Never consider yourself to be the cause of the results of your activities, nor be attached to inaction.

Dealing with ill health

1.A week before the exam

I had typhoid a week before my engineering entrance exam. Without much delay, I got admitted to hospital and got the best treatment possible, so that I will at least be able to show up at the exam center.

Try to recover before the exam. Stay optimistic. If unfortunate things happen, that is not the end of life. You will have another chance or go for a different career path.

2.A day before the exam

- If it is mild sickness, see a doctor and take measures for immediate relief
- If it is severe, it is okay to skip the exam. Health is more important than the exam

3.On the exam day

Go to the exam hall only if the body permits. A year lost doesn't cost your life. You are smart and you can make up for it.

Scheduling the exam

When to schedule the exam?

- If it is an exam where you have the choice of scheduling the date, plan for the exam date after you are comfortable with the basics
- Select the exam date based on how many holidays or leaves you get from work
- If your percentile depends on how many people take the test in that slot, go for a less sought out slot
- If you are someone who can learn the exam strategy from others, schedule for a later date in the window period
- If you are someone who gets more anxious after knowing the current exam pattern and can't wait till your turn comes, choose an earlier date
- If you are a girl who has a tough time during menstruation, choose a date far away from your date

☐

Chapter 13 - How to write the exam

After reading this chapter you will learn

- What to do on the exam day and in exam hall
- How to write subjective exams
- How to write objective exams

On the exam day

- Wake up on time
- Take bath even if you don't have the habit
- Meditate to calm your mind
- Don't skip breakfast
- Don't keep reading until the last minute. Most of it won't stick and will only add to exam stress
- Ensure that you are carrying all the items in your checklist
- Reach exam center at least 30 minutes before the scheduled time
- Check if the bench or computer is fine

In the exam hall,

Do

- Meditate before you get the exam paper
- Visualize doing well in the test
- Write your hall ticket number clearly
- Sign on the attendance sheets
- Keep sipping water
- If it is an objective paper, mark the answers on the OMR sheet periodically. Don't wait until the last minute. Be as careful while coloring as you are while solving the problem
- Read the questions clearly

- Check if there is a choice
- Attempt the required number of questions in the required number of words
- Check if the word is 'not' or 'except'
- Be extra careful when the options are
  - all of the above
  - more than one of the above
  - none of the above
  - can't be determined
- After you finish answering, if you have time at the end, recheck your answers. If it is a mathematical problem, try solving it in a different way and check if you are getting the same solution.
- Write as neatly as you can.
- If you have taken additional sheets, make sure that your name and hall ticket are written on them too. Tie the knot a little loose so that the papers can be turned without getting torn. At the same time, don't tie it too loosely that it unties by itself.

Don't

- Stare at the window
- Make eye contact with others
- Look for attractive people in the room
- Drink too much water
- Get stressed
- Strike off a lot in the paper. It gives a bad impression to the examiner.

Answering Subjective Papers

When you write subjective exams, remember that there is no single correct answer. What you write is open to interpretation by the examiner. If the examiner is impressed, you will be awarded more marks. Also, the examiner is a human, he also has bad days and bad moods. He wants his life to be easy.

Now keeping that in mind, what is the first thing which impresses the examiner?

1. Handwriting:

When I was in school, my teacher showed my paper to the entire class on how my handwriting makes my answer sheet look like a printed paper. If you don't have a good handwriting, working on improving it will definitely fetch you some extra points. A neatly written paper is a cake walk for the examiner. Even if you don't have time for improving it, you can improve the look of your handwriting by

- Writing medium sized on a ruled answer sheet
- Leaving enough space between lines and words
- Use two different inks. Write the headings in black and the content below it in blue or vice-versa
- Underlining the important points

2. Organise your answer

You might know the answer to the question but how you present it makes all the difference.

- Write the definition or introduction
- Outline the important terms
- Then explain them
- If required write examples for each

Use a differences table when question asks you to compare. If possible, draw a few flow charts here and there to make the paper look interesting.

3. Keep the word count in mind

Arrange the answer in terms of the number of words they are asking you to explain in. If it is below 100 words, get to the point directly. If it is around 500 words, write down the details. If it is more than that explain with examples.

4. Frame your answer based on what they are asking for

a) Explain

If you are supposed to explain rocket propulsion to a kid, you will not simply tell the definition and leave. You will start off with the basics and tell what a rocket is, how it works, what the parts of it are and then talk about rocket propulsion.

b) Examine

Imagine you are a civil engineer. You are told that building is deteriorated. Now you need to examine it to understand what caused the deterioration and how it can be fixed. So when you examine, you are digging deeper to find the underlying truth.

c) Describe

Here you get a chance to talk about the all the trivial details too as long as it adds value to answering the question. After you are done describing, even if the reader has never seen the object, he should be able to visualize it. That is the expectation out of describing.

d) Discuss

When you are asked to discuss, it is about evaluating it from all the angles. When you discuss a topic with friends, each one has their own point. So, you need to cover it in all angles and then conclude.

Which pen to use?

It is indeed painful to write at a stretch for 2 or 3 hours. The pen you select plays a major role along with what you have studied. But what factors matter in pen selection?

a) Finish on the paper:

Even though gel pens or ink pens give a nice look, make sure to use them only if they are waterproof. If they are not, what is the whole point in giving a neat look if the ink is going to be smudged? A few ball pens also give the finish of gel pens. Look out for different brands to know which one gives the best look.

b) Thickness of the pen:

Depending on your finger length and thickness, some prefer fat pens and a few others thin pens. Choose what works better for you. In case, you like the refill of a fat pen but like the thin pen, cut or add some stuff at the bottom of the pen you like to make the refill fit into it.

c) Grip:

Some pens have firm grip, sticky rubber grip, a few others smooth grip and a few with no grip at all. I can never write for a long time with a pen with no grip. When I was writing my subjective assignments recently, I realized that by changing the pen, I could change the number of hours I could sit at a stretch to write.

d) Smooth writing:

Sometimes, you want to keep writing because writing with the pen is smooth. That is the kind of pen you need to choose for exams.

e) Non-leakage:

The worst thing that can happen in the middle of the exam is a pen leaking and spoiling the answer sheet. You can either be a loyal user of the same pen for the entire year or take reviews from your friends about the same.

Should you start with the long or short answers?

If you are someone who might easily get tired and lose focus, you can start with the short ones first. It gives you a confidence of scoring a certain amount of marks. Then you can proceed further and answer the long ones.

If you are someone who knows answers to all the questions and can retrieve answers under stress too, start with long answers. Even if you run out of time at the last minute, you can scribble the answers for the short ones.

In what order should you answer the questions?

Ideally, answer them in the order asked in the question paper. It will make the life of the examiner easy. But if you are not sure of answers to all the questions, start with the one you are most confident about. This gives the first best impression to the examiner.

Of all the strategies mentioned above, which one should you follow?

Write a few mock tests. Try out different strategies. Go for the one which suits you the best. Even if you choose to answer the questions in random order, at least answer questions of the same section at one place to make it easy for the examiner.

Objective type – General Instructions

- Be extra careful with calculations when the answer options are very close
- If the answer options are far off, you can do approximations and educated guesses

- All, only, none, always are dangerous words. Make sure to pay extra attention when they are classifying it universally or specifically. Example: No mammal lays eggs. It is a false statement because Duckbilled Platypus does. So, whenever a universal classifier is there, recollect the exceptions.
- When it is a matching type of problem, don't solve the entire set. Work from the options and check only the controversial ones. For example, if the options are A) 1-b, 2-c, 3-a B) 1-c, 2-b,3-a C) 1-a , 2-b,3-c. You don't have to know about 1. Solve for 2 and 3.
- If it is an arranging type of question, the options tell you the order of a few statements. Make use of it for solving the test. For example, if the options are A) abcd B) cdab C) acdb D) acbd. In all the options you notice that b comes after a and d comes after c. That part of the question is solved for you. Compare if a or c comes first to proceed with the question.
- Be careful about the units. The question can be in thousands and the answer options in millions.

Objective -Specific type of questions

1.Reading Comprehension

a) Common misconceptions

- All the paragraphs need to be read
- All the questions need to be answered
- RC requires speed reading
- I need to make notes

b) Reality

- Sometimes all the answers can be in one para. Read only the parts of the paragraph which provide you the answer.
- You need to learn to be choosy. Answer the ones which are direct first.
- RC requires selective reading. Your speed does not matter. Comprehension is what matters.
- You need to note only what is required for the answer

c) **Approach**

Read the questions. Read the options. Sometimes you can eliminate the options without even reading the para. Now it gives you an idea on how to approach the para. Glance through the para and read slowly at the point which is going to answer the question.

d) **Common doubt**

"I am stuck with two options. How do I decide which one is correct?"

Collect proof for each option. For whichever option the proof is stronger, choose that one.

"It takes more than 10 minutes to read a para."

Don't read it all. Be selective.

e) **Common mistake**

Students get involved in the paragraph and get lost in thoughts. The para is there not to entertain you but to test you. You can entertain yourself outside the exam hall and not in the exam hall.

2. Vocabulary

a) Word roots

Check if you can break the word into two parts. Try to answer the meaning based on the individual words. For example, consider somnambulist. The word parts of it are somna and ambul and ist. The first part means sleep and the second is walking and the third part gives it the total meaning of the person who walks in sleep.

b) Context

Try to recollect if you have used that word in any other context before. Even if you don't know the word, you can guess the meaning of it. For example, Andrea agreed to meet today. We had a rendezvous as planned. Even if you don't know what a rendezvous means, in this context, you know that it has got something to do with the meeting.

If you can't figure out neither the word parts nor the context, it is always advisable to leave the question if it carries negative marking.

3. Data Interpretation

Rule no.1
If every set carries the same the number of marks, choose the one which is the easiest.

Rule No. 2
Just because you selected a data interpretation set, does not mean that you must solve all the problems in it. Choose the ones which are less time taking. You can leave the difficult ones for the last.

Rule No.3
Even if you don't have the time for the entire DI set, do the easiest one from the set.

Question Selection

The greater the number of questions you practice, the better you become in selecting questions. The type of questions you see in exams are
1. Questions which you already practiced
2. Questions you practiced but with a twist
3. Questions you practiced but different wording style
4. Questions of known concept but a different model
5. Questions with multiple concepts

Whatever the question is, you should be able to recognize it and classify it. If it is of the first type, you can jump and solve it. For the second type, if you can recognize the twist within a few seconds solve it or else you can leave it in case of a time crunch. For the third type, if you had practiced enough type of problems under each concept, you will be able to quickly recognize the wording style. The fourth type is a bit tough unless you have practiced thinking out of the box during preparation. The fifth will involve a couple of steps but you should be able to do fine.

So, if you are someone who studied only the basics, you should target getting all the type 1 right. If you are someone who practiced enough, you should focus on 3 and 5 along with 1.

If you have practiced well, you will be able to identify the trick of type 2 and with a little bit tuning, you can try 4 too.

The biggest trap none of you should fall into is spending too much time on type 2 and 4 trying to figure out what it is.

In case, you can see the entire question paper before you start solving and all questions carry equal marks, this trick is for you.

Classify the questions into easy, medium and tough.

a) Easy

- Known question and takes less time to solve
- Direct formula application
- Known solution

b) Medium

- Known question but can't recollect
- Need to do some steps before applying the formula
- Questions with multiple concepts

c) Tough

- Questions with a twist
- Questions with hidden known concepts

Don't attempt (in case of negative marking)
- Don't know the concept
- Don't know the formula

This methodology helps you prevent spending time unnecessarily on tough questions and losing out time in the end where you don't even look at the easy questions.

Does it not take a lot of time to classify?

While you go through the paper, attempt the easy questions simultaneously. So, you must ideally mark only the remaining type of questions. Also, by the time you finish the first round of going through the paper, you would have solved the easy questions which gives you the confidence to solve the remaining questions

If you want to use this strategy directly on the day of the exam, it might be unfruitful. Practice this on a few mock tests before you jump into it.

Which pen to use?

Online:

For online exams, you may not be allowed to take your own pens. This implies that it is a better habit if you had already learnt to write with all types of pens instead of having a pen of your choice

Offline:

This type of examinations usually involves OMR sheets where the bubbles must be colored. While in all other cases you look for a fine tip but it, in this case, use the one which has a blunt nib. Usually, the preferred color is black. Go to a store and check out the different types of pens. Shortlist a few and try a different one for a different exam. It is better to practice with this pen for your mock exams too so that you will know which pen you are more comfortable with.

Chapter 14 - What to do after the exam?

After reading this chapter you will learn

- How you should deal with your exam performance

One-time exam

Take an off. Relax. Make it your day, irrespective of how you did in the exam. If you did it well, feel optimistic about results but don't feel overconfident.

If you didn't do it well, no point in crying over spilled milk. Set some time for grieving but let it go after that. Analyze why you could not perform well.

- Was it the lack of conceptual knowledge?
- What are subject areas you didn't do well in?
- Were you not able to recollect the concepts?
- Which type of note making did you follow?
- Were you not able to apply the concepts?
- How well did you practice before the exam?
- Would solving more problems help you?
- Did you come across the same issue during your mock tests?
- Were you not able to manage the time?
- Did you follow the question selection strategy?
- Or was it exam stress?
    - What were the reasons behind your stress?
    - How can you eliminate those triggers?

Can you work on these weak areas to be well prepared for the next time?

Series of exams

Don't let your failure in one subject ruin your performance in the next subject. Each paper is independent. Forget that it happened. In JEE test, I would have done the second paper better if I had not let the feeling of not performing well in the first paper affect me. Now when I write CAT, I don't let my performance in one section affect my performance in the next section. A lot of students give up after they don't do well in one section which ruins their chances of success. What if the paper was tough and everyone else also didn't perform well? Each section is independent. You can't change the past but you can work in the future.

Block 4 - Becoming the topper

You now know how to gain subject knowledge and write an exam well. Even though a lot of students do all this, they still can't see any success. The problem comes due to attitude towards exams and life in general. The one thing which separates the students who top the exam from those who don't is optimism in life. The students who believe that their intelligence levels can be changed are more likely to succeed. Qualities you possess make a lot of difference in reaching your goals along with subject knowledge you possess.

"Your level of success rarely exceeds your level of personal development, because success is something you attract by the person you become." - Hal Elrod

Chapter 15 - Attitude

After reading this chapter you will learn

- The good attitudes to develop
- The bad attitudes to get rid of

The good

1. Be optimistic

Your explanatory style of events defines whether you are an optimist or pessimist which in turn defines your success in long-term. If you are an optimist, you look at failing in an exam as a one-time event. You think that it has got to do with external factors too and not your ability. If you are a pessimist, you think it is purely due to your inability. It will be a permanent event for you. Hence you will stop working hard for the next exam.

Next time, when a negative event occurs, notice your words. Are you considering yourself a failure? Or are you looking at it as a failed event? This change in speech helps you become and optimist.

2. Grit

"Hard work beats talent when talent doesn't work hard." - Tim Notke

You might not have an aptitude for an exam. But consistent efforts can get you there. I have a student who does terribly in class. He failed to get through the exam last year. But he enrolled for classes this year again. He makes a note of every small point I teach. He asks why he went wrong. He is a perfect example of grit. There are brighter students in my class than him. I know that even they will clear the exam with efforts. But this student puts additional efforts to become par with them. That makes a difference in the long term.

3. Growth mindset

A person with a growth mindset will never feel limited about his intellectual capacity. He will do whatever it takes to grow beyond what he is gifted with. Changing your belief that you can also top the exam by putting in efforts will make a lot of difference.

4. Deliberate practice

I practice the same exercise every day. The pain and strain which I feel on the first day, I no longer feel it on the 30th day. My body gets used to it. Practice made me perfect. But to lose more weight, I need to do something different.

Similarly, regular practice helps you become perfect with the basics. With practice, you move from 90 to 99. But to go from 99 to 100, you need to do deliberate practice. It is not about doing the default but about putting focused attention with an intention to increase the performance.

5. Delayed Gratification

The famous Stanford Marshmallow experiment, where children were offered two choices - an immediate small reward or a bigger delayed reward. When those children were tested at a later point of time, researchers noticed that those who were able to delay their gratification were a lot more successful academically than those who were not.

By delaying your gratification, you will be able to put in consistent efforts every day to see the result in your exams after long study sessions.

6. Cultivate the art of figuring out on your own

A lot of students do well as long as they are taught in a structured way. They score well in the exams too as long as the exam is tested on what they learned. But they can't deal with surprise elements. They go into a panic mode when they see something unexpected. This is because they don't have the skill of figuring out things on their own.
Students who possess this skill are those who are not afraid of failure. They try different methods without the fear of failing in them. They seek challenges to push themselves beyond the known comfort zone.

To develop this,

- Keep your curiosity alive and feed it.
- In your free time, do a research on a totally unrelated topic and present it in a crisp form
- Study lessons before your teacher teaches them
- Try solving puzzles. Even if you don't get the answer, it helps your problem approaching skills.

Once you start figuring out things on your own, you get a new sense of confidence to write any type of exam.

The bad

Characteristics of people who fail

1. You read but never practice

You keep reading day after day. In the end, you feel happy that the entire syllabus is done. But you never recall in between to see how much you remember.

Solution

For everything you read, write down a summary at the end of the day. Take periodical mock tests.

2.You are stuck in self-pity

You remind yourselves everyday how unlucky you are. You only feel sad that you were not born intelligent.

Solution

Accept that you can't change the factors which are not in your control. Play with the cards you are dealt with.

3.You give up on the face of slight difficulty

You start a new topic today. After a page, you find it difficult to understand. You give up and go for playing.

Solution

Break the concept into smaller parts. Take help of a friend or teacher to overcome the obstacle instead of abandoning the subject.

"Most of the important things in the world have been accomplished by people who have kept on trying when there seemed to be no hope at all."—Dale Carnegie

4.You don't do deliberate practice

You are happy to learn a concept. But you don't put any efforts to perfect it. As a result, you won't be able to do that problem in exam.

Solution

Whatever skill you choose, work on the intricate details of it. It is tough but it is worth the efforts.

5.You don't learn from mistakes

You make the same mistakes over and again because you don't care to take time out to review them.

Solution

Every time you make a mistake, do an analysis on why it happened, what could you have done differently to avoid it, what can you do now about it.

6.You don't convert your weakness to strengths

You keep avoiding the subjects you don't like only to end up with the entire syllabus to be studied in the last minute.

Solution

Be aware of the topics you are avoiding to study. Push it as a 10-minute study task at different points of the day. The ten minutes will add up to finishing the syllabus in the end.

7.You want to put one-night show

Studying the night, the final exam never helps. Successful students have a chain of daily routines which help them do well in exams.

Solution

List the routines you require to study for an exam.

The attitude which pulls you down in life is gossip, comparison, and envy.

1. Gossip

Gossip which started as a social bonding activity in the early days now ruins mental peace.

A few people gossip because that is the only way to make friends for them. When two people dislike the same person, they become thick friends. Their friendship runs on the hatred for the common enemy. Shared hatred makes a stronger bond than shared positivity. For a few others, it helps in overcoming their inferiority complex. Some do it out of envy. Whatever might be the reason for it, it is a negative behavior which pulls you down in life.

a) It lowers your value

"Great minds discuss ideas; average minds discuss events; small minds discuss people." – Eleanor Roosevelt

Don't be the small mind.

b) It lowers trust levels

No one trusts a person who gossips. People want their secrets to be safe. The person whom you gossip with will not trust you because he knows that you will gossip about him with someone else.

c) It ruins relations

People who gossip do not have healthy relations. Their relations live on negativity. They just live on a guilty pleasure. And all they have are superficial friends. Happiness depends on the number of quality friends you have and not quantity.

d) It breeds negativity

If you keep gossiping all the time, you are only looking at the negative qualities in a person. You will never be able to be happy if you continue your life in negative pleasure. When you look at the positive qualities in a person, life looks more positive.

e) It does not help you grow

When you satisfy your ego by gossiping, you are only looking for ways to put others down but not the ways in which you can improve. Do you want to keep degrading or improving in life?

How to not gossip?

a) Put yourself in other's shoes

Have you ever heard a gossip about you come back to you? How did you feel? You must have felt very humiliated. Won't other people feel the same? Irrespective of whether they are good or bad, you don't have the permission to hurt others. You have better work to do than judge others. If you truly think what they have done is wrong, inform the person what the right behavior is. Talking behind their back helps no one, including you and him.

b) Triple filter test by Socrates

Whenever you are tempted to gossip, ask the following three questions:
Is it true?
Is it good?
Is it useful?
If the answer is false even for one of them, don't talk about it.

c) Ask yourself "What's bothering me?"

When you feel like gossiping, ask yourself why you feel like gossiping. If your friend topping the exam is bothering you, work on doing well.

d) Make healthy relations

Develop a few hobbies. Read more about what interests you. Next time you meet your friends you can talk about interesting topics. Tell them what you learned in a way they can relate to. They will start liking you.

2.Comparing yourself to others

Ram and Shyam went to the same coaching center to prepare for GMAT. They discussed together and wrote the exam on the same day. Ram scored 740 while Shyam scored 670. Shyam was highly dissatisfied and went around telling people how Ram was lucky to get 740 even though both prepared together.

What does Shyam gain from this?

1. Sympathy for his loss
2. Make hard work of Ram look like luck

But what does it look like for others?

Shyam is feeling entitled.

I once had a friend who went around telling how her manager treats her like shit when compared to others in her team and how she deserves the best projects. It did not work. She used to talk the same way about every aspect of life. She was only comparing all the time.

I was so fed up after a certain time that I avoided going for lunch and snacks break with her.

What happens when you compare yourself to others?

1. You will sound entitled

Just like my friend, you will end up becoming a repelled. It feels annoying for people to hear your endless 'I am entitled' stories. You will also stop putting in efforts because you think you already deserve it.

2. People will avoid you

Your friends will understand that tomorrow you are going to compare yourself with them.

3. They think you are a loser

You don't become the champion by undermining others' efforts.

4. You will reduce your chances for success

When your focus is on others, you are losing out on the bigger picture- the strategy. Work on yours. If needed, copy their strategy shamelessly as long as it is not illegal.

5. Your scarcity mentality will grow

There is enough luck for everyone on the earth. Others getting what they want does not reduce your chances of working towards it.

6. You will feel more inferior

Whatever you focus on, it will magnify. If your focus is on why others got and not you, only that inferiority feeling magnifies. You are comparing in the first place because you want to prove that you are not bad. Comparing erodes your self-esteem.

What to do instead?

a) Are you ready to put in the same efforts?

Ram went home and put extra efforts for preparation. Shyam ignored that suggestion when Ram suggested. Does he have the right to compare now?

b) There is enough for everyone on the earth

Throw the scarcity mentality in the dustbin. Feel abundant. Congratulate your friend heartfully. Work on your path. Give your best.

3. Envy

Envy pulls you down. Hatred reflects hatred. You call others lucky and yourself unlucky. But if you evaluate it, you will find that it is totally wrong. You are only looking at the tip of an iceberg and not the entire iceberg. You do not know the various skills he has been putting in to reach the current position.

The ways to avoid jealousy

a) Learn from them

Next time you find yourself envious, question it. If your friend has topped the exam while you did not, think what could have been the reasons. Disturbing his studies, so that he doesn't do well in the exam won't help either of you. Learning techniques from his studying style and analyzing your poor strategies might help you step up to the next level.

b) Enjoy the process

You feel envy because you constantly worry about the end goal. When your friend tops the exam and you don't, the envy comes into picture. Instead, if you were enjoying the journey, without waiting for the destination to arrive, there is no scope for envy.

c) There are enough top ranks for every student

When I was in school, my teacher used to tell that she was ready to give the first rank for the all students of the class if all of us scored equally. But no one really cared to work hard for it. If your friend is doing well, you should not be envious about that. Instead, you should also work on doing better. The world needs the best people to make it a better place to live. Do you want to waste time feeling jealousy instead of being one of the best people on earth?

Chapter 16 - Habits

After reading this chapter you will learn

- How to develop a morning routine
- How to develop a evening routine
- Other good habits

Develop a morning routine

In my school days, my mom never switched on Television in the morning. She used to ask us to exercise for 5 minutes and then read the lessons for the day. Songs, TV, entertainment, arguments - none of these were allowed.

There lies my foundation of a morning routine. It had a significant effect on me.

Why do you need a morning routine?

When you wake up in the morning, your brain had already had at least 8 hours of rest. It is ready to take the best decisions and can grasp anything quickly. If that time is lost, the next best time if after a nap in the noon. But not everyone gets a chance to take a nap. And that is still not as effective as the morning time.

Morning Routines

Here is the entire list of things I did as a part of my morning routine during various times of my life. You can pick a few to start with.

1. Wake up without alarm

On any given day, I wake up without an external alarm. Only on the days, I have extremely important things to do, I use an external alarm too. But rest of the days, I tell my subconscious the previous day when it needs to wake me up. I was never able to leverage the power of subconscious mind this well in any other task. But for waking me up, it works wonderfully. You should give it a try.

In today's world, where there is no difference in day and night, I do agree that alarm has been one of the best inventions of mankind. But these alarms have been doing an equal level of harm to human wellbeing. When the alarm clock goes off in the morning, the day which has to start pleasantly will start with the release of stress/ fear, because you are being woken up by an external force. This in result produces negative chemicals in the brain. It is not about this. Sleep works in cycles of four stages. You will be in deep sleep in the third and fourth stage. It is during this stage the muscle is repaired and energy for the next day is built. If alarm rings when your sleep is in this stage, you feel fatigue the entire day even though you slept for entire 8 hours. It has been 2 years that I have stopped using an alarm. I use it only on the days when I am afraid of not waking up early. I feel fresh daily.

Start sleeping early. Try to tap into your subconscious mind and give instructions on when to wake up. Stop using the alarm for a week and see if the consequences are undesirable. If they are, probably your subconscious mind will start listening to you.

2. Affirmation

"Today is going to be a great day."
"I am going to study effectively today."
"I enjoy learning"

Prepare your own affirmations. Welcome the day on a positive note. Even if your day is going bad, affirmations infuse their positivity.

3. Diary dump

I don't remember my dreams or early morning thoughts in the later part of the day. So as soon as I wake up I write it in my diary, all my dreams and insights. Dreams tell a lot about your worries and concerns. If you sleep in the night thinking about a problem, you get insights about it the next morning.

Apart from this, you can also write about your worries for the day. This makes you a little calmer and more prepared for the day.

4. Mirror talk

Look into the mirror and make an eye-contact with yourself. "You will do it". That is all you need to say with a smile. It gives you a lot of confidence. You can add whatever you want to talk to yourself too.

5. Brush with left hand if you are a right-hander

Brushing with left hand will not only exercise the right part of the brain but also the brush reaches to parts of your mouth which your right hand can't reach.

6. Drink lukewarm water with lemon and honey

The best way to treat an empty stomach is to give it a glass of lukewarm water with lemon and honey. It will not only clean your stomach but also improves your metabolism.

7. Meditation

This is more about pranayama than about meditation. A few deep breaths will clear your respiratory tract and mind.

8.Cold water bath

Cold water pushes you out of your comfort zone. It makes you more alert.

9.Dress well

Dressing up well gives you more confidence. You will study with greater concentration. It is also known to pump up cognitive skills.

10.Healthy breakfast

Eat a protein-rich breakfast in the morning.

Develop a night routine

1.Spend time with family

Relationships make a lot of difference in your general temperament and the amount of success you achieve in life. A happy family life helps you beat the stress of the day and helps you develop strong bonds.

2.Be creative

All work and no play makes Jack a dull boy. Even though studying is important, you need ways to relax too. Find a creative outlet than watching television to discover yourself.

3.Reflect on the day

Think about what went well, what you could have done better and what you learned during the day.

Other Useful Habits

1. Drink enough water

Health is wealth. Even though it is a cliché. It needs to be called out as it has significant impact on your health.
When I was in school, my class teacher told us a story of a distant cousin of hers whose kidney failed because she forgot to drink water as she was busy with her research.
That one incident changed the amount of water I drink daily. I don't care where I am going, I always carry a water bottle with water in it with me.
When you are studying keep a water bottle beside you. It not only hydrates your body at regular intervals but also helps in reducing the stress levels. You need not worry about going to the restroom in between as it acts as a break and exercise you need.

2. Exercise

You read this everywhere. Yet I repeat it. Exercise daily. It does not matter for how long. But move your body.
One of the habits which my mom inculcated in me was to exercise every morning. In my school days, all I was expected to do was use a skipping rope and jump for some time. Or move my hands and neck for some time. Thankfully, even that counted as an exercise.
When I was 10, she introduced me to yoga. I found it more calming. But I could start practicing it full-fledged only after 14. That transformed my life in a way no other exercise did. The rebelling, annoyed and arrogant teenager became a lot calmer and easier to handle. I could notice the difference for myself.
In my twenties, I even tried walking, jogging and body weights. Jogging gave me new ideas for writing. Body weights increased my confidence levels. They taught me the importance of pushing myself a little more.

Why should you exercise?
- Provides you oxygen
- Improves your energy level
- Helps you focus better
- Releases endorphins which will keep you happier
- Helps you sleep better

Reasons why students don't exercise

a) "I wake up late. Exercise has to be done only in the morning."

I rarely wake up late. But it does not matter when I wake up. I still exercise. You sweat a little bit more due to the heat if you exercise late but it is fine as long as you are putting an effort towards exercising.

b) "I don't have time."

Do you rush to the class without brushing? Exercise is as important as brushing. You are not giving it the due the importance it needs to be given.

c) "I don't have to lose weight"

Exercise is not only for those who want to lose weight. It is for the mind too. A healthy mind resides in a healthy body. Take care of both. If you are afraid that calorie losing activities like running or weightlifting will make you thinner, go for yoga. My yoga master used to say that " Yoga is an exercise which will help the fat ones lose weight and the thin ones gain weight."

d) "I am lazy"

If you are lazy, the laziness will show up in your marks too.

What type of exercises to do?

You don't have to restrict yourself to only one type of exercise. You can try a variety of them and then stick to whatever is comfortable and suits your body type and schedule.

a) Stretch

This is the easiest. Long hours of studies hurt your neck and lower back. Flexing your muscles during study breaks will prevent the pain.

b) Walk

All you need is a pleasant environment to go for a walk. You can either go alone or with a study mate. If you are alone, recollect the concepts or think about pleasant things in life or just stay in the present and observe the people around you. If you are with your study mate, you can discuss the concepts. Even if you just let the mind wander, it helps in divergent thinking which connects the disparate concepts.

c) Jog

If you feel that walking is for old people, you can jog. This will help you to breathe a little deeper.

d) Yoga

This is one of the best exercises to do. It will take some time and might require you to spend some money to get trained under a yoga master. Even though there are a lot of videos on the internet, it is advisable to learn it from an expert who checks your postures before you start doing it on your own.

e) Body weights

Unlike gym, you don't need any equipment for it. Your body is the tool. If you are looking for an improvement in your confidence or a way to channel your anger or aggression, this is the way to go.

f) Skip

All you need is a skipping rope. Start jumping.

g) Gym

As a student, you might not be able to afford spending amount on a gym membership. But if you can, take care that the exhaustion won't keep you away from studies.

h) Aerobics

It will be fun and easy.

i) Dance

If you don't want to go anywhere or lazy to do any exercise, you can play some music and jump. It will be both entertaining and exercising.

3. Sleep well

a) Number of hours of sleep

A few pieces of research say that 8 hours sleep is required. A few more say that it does not matter how many hours you sleep. You should feel comfortable with the amount of rest. From my experience, sleep is the best medicine you can have any time. You need enough rest for the neurons to remove the toxic material and consolidate whatever you studied during the day.

b) Sleep timings

This again depends on your comfort zone. I won't say that you must wake up at 5. Irrespective of when you wake up, if you stick to your study schedule, you will do fine.

c)Naps

It is an art to be able to take a power nap. It will provide you the rest you require in between studies. But then if you are not a power nap type of person you are still fine.

Afternoon naps-

It is difficult to concentrate after lunch. The energy in the body gets diverted to the digestion of the food instead of letting the brain have it. It is okay to sleep in the noon as long as you don't sleep for a really long time which affects your schedule.

4.Write a Journal

Tracking your day helps you understand how you have been progressing in your life in general and with your studies in particular. It can act as your goal tracker. Write down your goals. Pin that page on the top. Every time you visit it, it keeps reminding you of them.

How to start writing a diary?

a) Online/ Offline or Soft copy/ Hard copy:

Decide that first. A lot of people fret over privacy. I suggest Evernote or WordPress private blog for these writers. At the other end of the spectrum are the writers who press on writing with a pen on paper. You can go for a diary with a lock or lock your diary in a safe place.

b) Time of the day:
A lot of them don't write because they forget or feel tired at the end of the day. So, decide when you want to write. Keep a reminder till it becomes a habit. The best way to write is whenever you think you want to share something for yourself.

What to write?

a) What did you do today?

It is the easiest diary prompt. At the end of the week, if you are doing the same thing every day, at least for the sake of writing something interesting in the diary you will want to change your routine.

b) Gratitude journal

Write down three things for which you are grateful today. Easy to write. It also improves happiness in the long run.

c) Goals

Once you are comfortable with the easy prompts, go a step ahead, discuss your goals with diary. Even ten years down the line it is going to make a lot of difference.

Review your diary periodically. See if you are making any progress in your goals. What is stopping you from achieving them? Can you do something about changing them?

5. Make use of your commute time

a) Meditation

My friend meditates while she commutes. She goes to college with a fresh mind. She focuses better. Her productivity levels are high. It is one of the best ways to make use of productive time because you might not be ready to spend time on meditation otherwise.

b) Visualization

While meditating, visualize yourself focusing well in the classes. If it is during exams, visualize that you are writing exams with full concentration.

c) Journal

You can write down your happy moments and stress points of the day to reflect on how the day went.

d) Learn new words

Commuting is the best time for rumination. You can learn a word and imagine it in different ways.

e) Play games

Not candy crush. Play brain games like crosswords, sudoku, etc. Something to train your brain.

f) Talk to people around you

If you are commuting with your parents, spend time with family. If you are going by a school or college bus, discuss the subject. If you are taking a public transport, learn about what is taught in other schools or colleges.

g) Mental Math

Once an MBA aspirant told me that he uses his commute time in doing mental math. That helped him increase his calculation speed and helped him land in a top B-school. All he did was revise tables, multiply and add whatever numbers he saw on the boards on the road. Isn't it simple?

h) Sleep

I envy those who can fall asleep as soon as they get on to a moving vehicle. That is the best thing to do while commuting.

6. Mind games/Puzzles

One day, my class teacher, who I thought was a very intelligent person, expressed her concern in the class that she was not able to solve Sudoku. I felt a childish accomplishment that I achieved something great because I could solve 5-star sudoku.

How do the games help you?

a) Logical intelligence:

Any person who does not have subject knowledge but can think logically can play these games. They activate the logical part of the brain. There are nine types of intelligence and logic is one of them. So you become logically intelligent as that part of your brain is getting trained daily.

b) Competitive exams:

When I was preparing for competitive exams, I could do linear and circular arrangement questions quickly. My friend took a lot of time to solve them. She thought I was blessed with logical intelligence. But the truth was I spent more time in training that area of my brain.

Inspite of the above, they don't help you crack exams. Because

i) It trains only one part of the brain.
ii) You need to establish connections in your brain to leverage this intelligence to solve other logical problems

My friend who cleared one of the toughest exams in India, can't solve a Sudoku of level beyond 2 of 'The Hindu paper' while I who could not clear the same exam can solve level 5 of Sudoku.

So don't expect magic to happen by solving puzzles.

7. Keep your brain sharp and active

a) Question everything

You see something weird, question it. I saw a traffic policeman dancing today. Numerous thoughts ran in mind about his behavior. What is making the policeman dance on a busy road? Is he entertaining others? Is he a mock policeman? Is there something about him on the news? Let it be anything. If they are activities, question why they should be done only that way. If it is people, think what ran in their mind to behave the way they did.

b) Create

Let it be a piece of prose or poetry or a simple drawing. Or if you are a music player, compose music. Whatever it might be, just create it. Don't care about how it comes out. It can take the worst possible shape, but still create it. Creation has a totally different effect on the brain from what consumption has.

c) Exercise & Meditation

I feel lazy when I don't exercise. Exercise keeps your day active when you do for optimal time. Deep breathing helps you better with oxygen supply which in turn helps in keeping the brain active.

d) Eat food on time

Brain constitutes only 2% of the body weight but consumes 20% of the energy. Don't let the brain down by consuming irregular meals.

e) Stop depending on calculator

When you are in the grocery store, calculate the approximate bill. When you are checking the distance, you need to travel further, calculate the percentage of distance you have traveled so far. Let it be anything. Give your brain a chance to calculate before you open your calculator.

f) Read

It expands your mind and helps you form new connections. The new concept you read today runs in the backend for the rest of day. Which in turn gives you new ideas to implement in your life.

What should you avoid?

a) Gossip

The negative talk about the third person feels so tempting but it drains all your energy. Avoid it at all costs.

b) Negative self-talk

Self-pity feels comfortable. But it deteriorates your brain. All the good habits you have go down the drain with this one habit.

c) Watching senseless TV serials and movies

Your brain ruminates on what you feed it. From where will you actively think about the material you studied if the stories of the soaps you watch take up the working memory?

d) Sitting idle

A short break after a focused session is useful to activate creative thinking. But long idle breaks make you dull. Indulging in activities which you love also constitutes rest. Stop acting like you need to sit idle for taking rest. If you feel the urge to sit idle, either meditate or sleep in corpse posture. But not an idle brain.

8. Improve your thought process

Another trick which comes in handy to improve your problem-solving skills is to improve thought process.

a) Question the existing thoughts

You don't have to do an extensive research on improving the thought process. You don't have to purchase additional material either. All you need to do is just change the perspective. Why should a carrot be used only as a vegetable? Why can't it be used as a fruit?

b) Copy the thought process

What is the approach used by the topper in solving the problem? The more you see smart techniques to solve a problem, the more you can learn to think like them.

c) Expand your mind

Read books and do courses which will challenge your thinking. A new perspective will make you creative and enhances out of box thinking.

d) Expose yourself to new surroundings

Occasionally go on a trip. If you can't do that, change your place in school/college. If that also can't be done, exchange your bedroom with that of your roommate/sibling. Or the simplest, change the direction of your sofa or table. Move the apps in your phone. Change your wallpaper daily. Any small change will also help in improving the thought process.

Bad habits

1. Trap of notifications

Why bad notifications are bad?

Have you noticed that when you learn a new word, you will start seeing that word everywhere?

Similarly, when you start your day with negativity, you will be seeing more of negative happenings throughout the day. Not that your day becomes negative, but your focus shifts to negative activity.

Why good notifications are bad?

Good notifications give you a rush of goodness. It sets your day to 'bring it on more' mode. When you don't get them more, you will start feeling frustrated and depressed. Since your mind is craving for it subconsciously, you can't focus fully on any task.

Now that we have come to an agreement that notifications are bad for our health, how can we avoid them first thing in the morning?

I have previously tried these, and they gave me wonderful results.

a) Close all the conversations in the night

If you are waiting for a text from the previous night, you are more likely to check the notification on phone.

b) Notifications from social media

What others are up to in their life is none of your business when it comes to priorities in life. How much others love you on social media also does not determine what you have to do today. So, it does not make any sense at all to check these notifications.

What to do instead?

a) Dump your thoughts

Brain gets good rest in deep sleep. You might get solutions for your problems during that rest time. Even if not for that, you can dump your early morning anxieties. When I start writing the first thing in the morning, I write about the dreams which I got in sleep. Dreams usually tell a little about our concerns in life.

b) Read a book

I read a book so that I get the same happiness that prior ones gave. One idea in the morning will bring a lot more ideas during the day.

2.'I am tired' excuse

After a long day, you go home and say this excuse every day. We are not tired. It is just an excuse we tell ourselves to not do any more productive work for the day. Do you feel the same when you must go home and meet your best friend after a long time? You feel the energy which you never had on normal days. Have you seen a kid who jumps all day, plays all day and still has the same energy when you come back home? Because they are doing what they enjoy. Even I used to go home and rest on sofa every day giving the 'I am tired' excuse. One day, I decided to stop telling this to myself and started reading as soon as I got home. It made a lot of difference in getting the momentum.

3.Letting others tell you that you can't do it

There is a famous story of a few frogs who accidentally slipped into a deep pit. All the frogs were trying to come out, but people outside were telling the frogs that the pit is deep, and they can't come out. All the frogs gave up except for one. It successfully came out because it was deaf and could not hear what people were saying. In fact, it thought that people were encouraging it to come out. Similarly, in daily life, a lot of people will tell you that you can't do a lot of things. It is you who should decide if it is worth trying and go for it even if people tell you that you are not capable of it.

4.Using Mobile phones in bed

Mobile phones are bad both before going to sleep and after waking up in the morning. The light emitted from the mobiles disrupts the sleep cycle. The buzzing sound does not let you fall asleep. The awaiting of notification keeps your brain alert. Overall, it is the worst thing to use if you plan on sleeping early.

When you wake up in the morning, your mind is fresh from a deep night's sleep. The ideas you get in the morning can be life changing. Instead of letting the mind give you those thoughts, you dump it with notifications from your smartphone again.

☐

Chapter 17-People

After reading this chapter, you will learn

- How to deal with parenting mistakes
- What type of people to have
- What type of people to avoid

Parenting mistakes

a) Money

If parents constantly complain about lack of money to spend on your education, it is a tough state to concentrate on studies. But on any day if you are attentive in class, you can earn a bit of pocket money by teaching weaker students.

b) Joint family

If the house is always crowded with people, it is tough to make space and find time to study. In that case, find a library or make friends with someone who is studious. Go home only after you are done studying for the day.

c) Household responsibilities

My mom never let me do the household work. She would tell me "Finish studying for the day. Then you are free to do whatever you wish to."

If the household responsibilities are a lot, it will be tough to make time for studying. But while doing the routine chores, instead of letting your mind wander, you can recollect your lessons.

d) Pressure

Criticism

It is painful to have parents who constantly tell you that you are useless. You can't stop them from expressing their fear. Instead of taking it at face value, understand that it is their way of emphasizing that you need to study. They have no intentions to hurt you. That is their way of motivating you.

Constant comparison

This is another ineffective way used by parents to motivate you. Instead of harboring negative feelings towards your friends or parents, take the deeper meaning and focus on becoming better

Pushing too hard

A few parents make their children wake up early in the morning and force them to study till late in the night. If your parents are like that, have an honest talk with them. Make it clear that you can't focus beyond a level and deserve a decent amount of sleep and should be able to enjoy studying.

Strict rules

The more a parent prevents you from watching the TV or using a smartphone, the more you will be drawn towards it. Make sure that you convey it to your parents and get into an agreement on the reasonable amount of entertainment which can be allowed.

People you need

1.Mentor

A mentor is a person who provides constructive criticism and pushes you beyond your comfort zone. When your peers tell you that you are doing well, they know it only by your marks. It's a compliment based on how you stand in comparison to them. But you need someone who can judge you by your true potential.
Even though mentors might sound harsh at times, you need that admonishing to score full marks in the exam. You should not worry if they keep pointing out your mistakes, but you should when they stop pointing them.

Randy Pausch, author of the Last Lecture aptly says this-
 "When you're screwing up and nobody says anything to you anymore that means they've given up on you...you may not want to hear it but your critics are often the ones telling you they still love you and care about you and want to make you better."
Mentors are not only there to give you feedback. They exist to help you avoid the mistakes which you are prone to make. They don't let you fall into the common pitfalls.

How to find your mentor?

Even though I was lucky to have a mentor at most of the stages of my life, I did not approach them. They wanted to mentor me because they saw the potential in me. Similarly, when you start putting in efforts, you will notice that teachers will want to help you. They will want to see you grow.
Paulo Coelho tells the same in Alchemist -
"And, when you want something, all the universe conspires in helping you to achieve it."

But if you want to start off with something and have no clue, approach the teacher who you want to be your mentor and ask specific questions. One of my students asked me how he should study to avoid the mistakes he has been making in the exams. I have been taking extra efforts to follow up with him since then as I saw the burning passion he has to do well in exams. He got a mentor by asking for it.

What should you not expect from a mentor?

Mentor is there only to guide you. Don't expect him to spoon feed you.

You are the one who is ultimately accountable for what you are doing with your life. You should not put the blame on your mentor for not guiding you all the time.

2.Accountability partner

2012

I told my mother - "Mom, I want to join a CAT coaching center"

2013

I told my friend - "You should join a coaching center for Civil services preparation."

2014

Friend asked - "Can you shift to my hostel? We shall study together."

2015

Study mate - "Send me the study plan. Let's stick to it."

2016

Friend asked - "You have not been writing these days?"

2017

Friend - "You are going to pay me Rs.100 every time you break the challenge."

2018

I said, " I am going to finish writing this book by April end."

None of the above goals would have been possible without the accountability.

Why do you need an accountability partner?

1. Stick to schedule

You are good with subjects. But you need a proper schedule to stick to it. A coaching center might help you with a study plan. Combined studies with the right group force you to stick to the schedule.

2. Motivation

If you are looking for external motivation, an accountability partner will help you with it. Every time you don't feel like doing, there is a person who is going to question you. A friend of mine asked me to keep asking him if he has studied or not every day. I have been asking him as a reminder and he feels forced to do it.

3. Guilt Trip

When you promise to study and don't study, won't it make you guilty that you are not able to keep up with your promise?

4. Make you keep going forward

Accountability partner challenges you into something every now and then. You will have to accept the challenge which in turn sets you onto a fast track mode.

How to find an accountability partner?

1. Online groups
There are tribes on many websites where the members of each tribe hold each other accountable for the progress they are making. They also post questions for discussion and doubts.

2. Join communities
A like-minded group fosters growth. Join a community where you will enjoy studying.

3. Friend
If you have a friend who is already doing well, you can ask him to be an accountability partner. When my friend asked me to be her accountability partner, both of us studied even more seriously than before.

Mistakes in selecting an accountability partner

1. Approach a person online who you think is doing well

The person you reached out to might be the best in your field. But he has his own life, priorities, and commitments. He must have even had his own mentor and accountability partner too. Why should he be your accountability partner?

2. Ask a person who has the capacity to hurt you

Accountability is about discipline. But discipline need not necessarily be in a negative way. He can make you pay for the missed schedules, but he should not taunt you and make you feel low about yourself.

3. Ask a random friend

I once had this friend as an accountability partner. I went to her place over the weekend to study. But all we did was cook, eat and sleep. I decided not to go to her place any time again for studying. Because she was not serious about it in the first place.

How to set the rules?

1. Agree on the schedule

I agreed to check on my friend if she was writing her mock tests or not every week.

2. Explain the task/activity/challenge clearly

"I challenge you to study one chapter daily. Reading it won't suffice. You should consolidate it in few sentences or a flowchart." In this case, the rules of the challenge are clear.

3. Agree on the consequences

My friend challenged me to run every day for 90 days. In case I miss any day, the challenge will start from the beginning again.

Copyrights

Copyright © Nikitha Mangu
All rights reserved. No part of this book may be reproduced in any form or by any electronic or mechanical means, including information storage and retrieval systems, without written permission from the author, except in the case of a reviewer, who may quote brief passages embodied in critical articles or a review. Trademarked names appear throughout this book. Rather than use a trademark symbol with every occurrence of a trademarked name, names are utilised editorially, with no intention of infringement of the respective owner's trademark. The information in this book is distributed on an "as is" basis, without warranty. Although every precaution has been taken in the preparation of this work, neither the author nor the publisher shall have any liability to any person or entity concerning any loss or damage caused or alleged to be caused directly or indirectly by the information contained in this book.

CPSIA information can be obtained
at www.ICGtesting.com
Printed in the USA
BVHW070938141021
618949BV00007B/88